Answer for Cancer: 9 Keys

B Mark Anderson

Answer for Cancer: 9 Keys

B Mark Anderson

What Others Are Saying

What an awesome story! This book is RIPE with powerful information that the world needs!

According to the most accurate research to date from Cancer Research UK and the British Journal of Cancer, one in two people will develop cancer at some point in their lives. When it comes to cancer (and all health conditions for that matter), always remember this: God has given your body the remarkable ability to prevent and heal cancer.

In this book, Mark Anderson outlines with eloquence a powerful mental, physical and spiritual approach to building a robust body, a steadfast faith and an overcomer spirit. Mark faced his cancer head-on and beat it by relying on lifestyle principles grounded in science and faith in the healing power of Jesus Christ. Now, he has been called to inspire and empower others to live life at a higher and a deeper level and heal the way God intended. This is a must read!

Dr David Jockers DC, MS, CSCS

In the age of quick fixes and too-easily concluded answers that often end up in failure, Mark takes the reader with him on his journey of the unexpected, shocking, sometimes fearful news of having the life-taking killer disease of cancer. Mark's experience opened my eyes and gripped my heart as I read of the torments he suffered in both mind and body.

Mark carefully pursued the Biblical and medical pathway to a joyful and successful victory. The Lord has indeed inspired Pastor Mark to write this book to glorify God and to walk others to health and healing through the cross of Jesus Christ and a healthy lifestyle.

We enjoyed the book so much and can't wait to give it to friends.

Bobby Martz, Founder of Hour of Harvest

I was stunned, first of all by all the suffering he had gone through, and second by what I had just read. I thought I was fairly knowledgeable about the care of the body. Wrong! He took me through a well-planned seminar in the first twelve chapters. Mark walked the tightrope of acknowledging the medical world for saving his life plus demonstrating the inescapable truths from alternative and nutritional medicine that keep him breathing.

I was fascinated (and taken back to high school chemistry) with subjects like detox and alkalization. Mark is not sloppy with the facts. He did careful research and presents it tastefully and often humorously. Then in the next part he led me into a refresher course in meditation, choosing key scriptures and highlighting truths such as the healing power of the cross. So we went from a medical/nutritional journal to a devotional guide, both parts rich in their own way. His book is believable and practical. It could change the way you do life. Did for me!

Paul Anderson, Director of Lutheran Renewal Services (Ret)

Answer for Cancer: 9 Keys is a resourceful and uplifting book in which Author/Pastor Mark Anderson comes alongside the reader with the warmth and encouragement any cancer patient and his family needs on this very difficult journey. Having "been there and done that," Pastor Anderson shares from his personal, real-life experiences and wisely balances three main areas of dealing with cancer: medicine, faith, and natural remedies. *Answer for Cancer: 9 Keys* will provide much insight to anyone … regarding cancer treatment as well as a gift of encouragement to others.

Pastor Jairo Carbajal, La Casa de mi Padre; Monterrey, Mexico

Very informative and researched well. I use some of the same alternative options to maintain my health. I highly recommend this book to grow spiritually as well as to greater understand the healing power that is available.

John Kummerfeld, cancer survivor since 2007

Answer for Cancer: 9 Keys is filled with information on how to fight and prevent cancer and it will definitely build your faith in God. And even if you don't believe in God, this book can help you win over cancer. It is plum full of nutrition and wellness information. Mark proves here that healing of cancer is possible for you as it was for him.

Read this book to find out how Mark won over inoperable Stage 4 lymphoma cancer.

Answer for Cancer: 9 Keys is loaded with hope and information for healing of bodies and minds. It can bring good or better health to all who read it. Here's help for people who are struggling with other health issues as well, not just cancer. Mark shares with the reader about his fight back to good health and the findings of his research for answers that can benefit many.

Greta Eubanks

Other Books by B Mark Anderson:

Local Churches, Global Apostles: How Churches Related to Apostles in the New Testament Era and Why It Matters Now—Ground-breaking research and surprising conclusions offer fresh perspectives on apostles and elucidate why the early church exploded with growth.

Eggnog Recipes: Eggnog Lore and Recipes Galore—Experience the fascinating history and health benefits of non-alcoholic eggnog throughout the centuries. Over 50 original eggnog recipes, organized month by month, will enthrall you year 'round.

Chicken Evangelism (forthcoming)—To register for a copy, contact the author at www.ChickenEvangelism.com

Contact the author at www.bmarkanderson.com

© 2016 B Mark Anderson

ISBN: 1533393702

ISBN-13: 978-1533393708

All rights reserved. No part of this book may be reproduced, stored in a retrieval system, or transmitted in any form or by any means, electronic, mechanical, photocopying, recording, or otherwise without written permission except in the case of brief quotations embodied in critical articles and reviews. For information or permission contact B Mark Anderson, 1575 Underwood Avenue, Muscatine, IA 52761.

> Edited by: Kari Anderson, Bethany Anderson, and Alison S. Britton
> Layout: Samuel Anderson and Alison S. Britton Consulting Services, Inc.
> Cover photo: Sarah Anderson

Unless otherwise noted, all Scriptures are from the New American Standard Bible (NASB) Copyright © 1960, 1962, 1963, 1968, 1971, 1972, 1973, 1975, 1977, 1995 by The Lockman Foundation. Where other translations are used, they are direct quotes with permission attribution recorded at the end of the book. No effort was made to correct grammar, punctuation, and spelling of the various translations except where needed to promote common sense understanding.

Notice of Medical Disclaimer: This book is intended for educational purposes. It is not intended to provide medical advice or to take the place of medical advice and treatment from your personal physician. Neither the publisher, nor the author, nor the author's ministry take any responsibility for any possible consequences from any action taken by any person reading or following the information in this book.

Every human individual differs from all others. No conventional or alternative treatment is guaranteed to produce health. Do not use this information if you are not willing to assume the risk. Always consult your physician, nutritionist, or other qualified health care professional before undertaking any change in your physical protocols, whether fasting, diet, medications, or exercise.

Foreword

To introduce myself, I have been Mark's physician since November of 2012 and a medical oncologist for nearly 30 years. As a typical general medical oncologist, certainly my focus of treatment has been by traditional medical therapies such as chemotherapy, radiation therapy, and other usual medical treatments; and that still remains my main focus.

However, like most cancer doctors who have been in practice for some time, I have developed an appreciation and admiration for less orthodox methods that patients have been able to incorporate into their care. Originally my focus was on my own successes and times that I felt that I had effected a cure, but as a very legitimate side track it has been very rewarding noticing that sometimes patients have done well beyond what I would have expected I could have achieved.

Of course, just as in traditional treatment, this is not always the case, and in many cases patients have obviously tried very hard and not done well despite theirs and their physicians' best efforts. Nevertheless, there is truly something to Mark's feelings and approach and over time it has become an enjoyable part of my practice. As in many facets of life, I have found bits of wisdom in his book that I do feel will come up at unexpected times and be very helpful.

As a tribute to Mark and his family, I would like to note a not uncommon, but nevertheless notable trait that he shares with many of my cancer patients. I am always impressed that Mark would always make a big effort to be gracious and considerate even when things were not going so well and he was not feeling very well. I, myself, find that I am not as thoughtful as I should be when I have been stressed by life's hurdles. I have always been amazed with how patients like Mark make such an effort to be kind to their family and caregivers. It is very much noted and appreciated and says a great deal about the person and the family/spiritual situation they came from.

Dr James Feeley, MD

Preface

"You have cancer"—the three most terrifying words you can hear. Why? Because the modern cancer treatments just don't work. Most people today realize this, thus fear follows a cancer diagnosis. However, despite the failure of modern treatments, as soon as you're diagnosed, the oncologist will likely recommend chemotherapy, radiation, and perhaps surgery.

The main issue with these "Big 3" treatments is that they all either cause cancer or facilitate the metastasis (spreading) of cancer. Over the past decade, I cannot count the number of cancer patients that have contacted me after doing a few rounds of chemotherapy and radiation and told me that their doctor initially told them "You're cancer free," only to have to break the bad news a few months later that "the cancer is back with a vengeance."

This is exactly what happened to Pastor B Mark Anderson, a happily married husband and father of 7 children, who began to have chest and stomach pains in 2011 and went to the doctor for some tests. Then he heard the three words—"You have cancer." After six rounds of chemotherapy, which Anderson calls "hell on earth," he was told that all tests indicated he was "cancer free."

But after only 30 days, an MRI indicated a new tumor in his lung. The cancer was back. Maybe it never left? Regardless, the doctor told Anderson that he only had a 10% chance with chemotherapy. Huh? The prognosis went from "cured" to "doomed" within 30 days. The reality is that much of what we've been taught about cancer and its treatments (and medicine in general, for that matter) isn't factually true. It's based on medical mythology grounded in corporate interests, including the drug companies ("Big Pharma") that want to sell you a dozen prescription medications and medical institutions that want you to remain a long-term repeat customer for life.

To achieve these profit interests, Big Pharma and medical institutions have devised a seductive mythology that has been pounded into the consciousness of consumers everywhere. This folklore includes some real whoppers such as "cholesterol causes heart attacks." But it's even more insidious than that. One of the most dangerous lies is the false idea that you are born "deficient" in chemotherapy, and that the only way you can cure cancer and be a normal, healthy human being is to subject your body to endless, high-profit interventions that just coincidentally happen to keep you sick and actually cause cancer, while keeping Big Pharma and the doctors very wealthy.

God opened Anderson's eyes to the reality that the chemotherapy would likely kill him, so he began to explore other options, and that's when he discovered Webster Kehr and www.CancerTutor.com. That was the day that the tide turned. That was the day that hope returned. That was the day that the Lord began to take him down the path of true healing.

Anderson began to mine the Scriptures for hope-filled and healing verses, as well as educate himself and his family about real treatments for cancer—not the false, deceptive treatments that are prescribed on a daily basis to millions of cancer patients worldwide. He began a journey to learn all he possibly could about cancer.

Answer for Cancer: 9 Keys, by Pastor Anderson, takes you on this breathtaking journey and will inspire and encourage you. On this journey, the author learned that the true contribution of chemotherapy to a 5-year survival rate is an abysmal 2.1%. He also learned about proven science-based cancer treatments, like alkalization and oxygenation, and about the importance of supporting the immune system, nutrition, and detoxification. You'll learn about the natural and spiritual keys to defeating cancer and will also learn about various Biblical methods that God uses to heal.

This book is a must read for you and your loved ones as it eloquently communicates information about the mental, spiritual, and physical attributes necessary to overcome cancer and live a long, healthy life.

Read it, follow it and free your mind and spirit.

God bless you all.

Ty M. Bollinger
Author of *Cancer—Step Outside the Box*
Producer of *The Truth About Cancer—A Global Quest*

Table of Contents

Part One—Death Came Knocking on My Door **1**

Part Two—Cancer is a Formidable Foe: Nine Natural and
Spiritual Keys for Prevention and Cure **13**

Chapter 1   First Key: Get a Coach **15**

Chapter 2   Second Key: See You Later, Meditator **21**

Chapter 3   Third Key: Love Can Save Your Life! **25**

Chapter 4   Fourth Key: Modern Medicine: Mixture of Miracle
            and Murder **27**

Chapter 5   Fifth Key: Oxygenation: We "Otto" Know by Now **31**

Chapter 6   Sixth Key: Be Wise—Alkalize! **37**

Chapter 7   Seventh Key: Marshall the World's Greatest Army:
            Your Immune System **41**

Chapter 8   Eighth Key: Diet, Nutrition, and Cooking:
            Who's in Charge—Mouth or Mind? **47**

Chapter 9   Ninth Key: Detox or Die—Slogan for the 21st Century **55**

Chapter 10 Summary: Here's What I Do **61**

Part Three—Meditation on God and His Word **65**

Chapter 11 God's Word is His Medicine **67**

Chapter 12 God Heals You by His Word **71**

Chapter 13 God Heals You by the Cross **75**

Chapter 14 God Heals You by His Spirit **81**

Chapter 15 God Heals You by Destroying the Devil's Works **85**

Chapter 16 God Heals—It's His Nature to Heal You **93**

Chapter 17	God Heals—It's His Pleasure to Heal You	**105**
Chapter 18	God Heals You Through Repentance	**113**
Chapter 19	God Heals You Through Faith	**117**
Chapter 20	God Heals You Through His Covenant	**125**
Chapter 21	God Heals You Through the Eucharist (Holy Communion)	**131**
Chapter 22	God Heals You Through Peace	**135**
Chapter 23	God Heals You Through Love and Compassion	**139**

Epilogue and Concluding Thoughts	**143**
Postscript	**149**
Acknowledgements	**155**
Additional Resources	**159**
Permissions	**163**

Part One

Death Came Knocking on My Door

No one needs to die from cancer. Nine keys—some natural, some spiritual—are woven into my recovery. With the aid of these nine, I won the cancer battle, and you and your loved ones can win it too. Here's my story.

God has spared my life several times. By His mercy, I have survived a plane crash and head injuries from falling out of a barn. I have survived a car accident and blood poisoning. God brought me safely through a river just a few feet above a raging cataract. I survived typhoid fever. And in Mexico, I was so sick from some form of "Montezuma's Revenge" that I prayed to die.

In spite of all this, or maybe because of these things, cancer was something I never expected. I have never smoked. (I tried it once as a boy with my neighbor's encouragement. We rolled up dried maple leaves in cardboard and I stuck the "cigarette" in my mouth. "Now suck in," my neighbor advised, and I complied. You guessed it—I seared my lungs. After that, I never tried again.)

The First Signs

Chest and stomach pains first began in 2011. The feelings were slight at first. I also had a slight numbness in my right foot. Since the chest distress was unremitting, I finally yielded to our family's requests; I went to the doctor. Dr. S., like any good doctor, examined me and ordered a treadmill test. The test was a breeze and the doctor quit the test early. "He has a perfect heart!" announced the doctor to all the surrounding attendants.

Since pastors often preach about the need for a pure heart, I can joke, "I'm a pastor with a perfect heart." I was 100% confident my heart was not a problem. I could ride a bicycle up hills as well as a teenager. My hobby is wood chopping and I could chop wood better than anyone I knew. I could have told the doctor my heart was fine by going for a walk with him.

More tests ensued. One MRI on my lungs showed minor spots. Since I farm as well as pastor a church, cancer specialists at the University of Iowa Hospital suspected I had "farmers' lungs," and suggested I come back for another checkup in six months. "Small spots on farmers' lungs are a reaction to soil conditions in Iowa and are not considered a problem," the doctor explained.

Eight months later, I underwent more tests. I was slowly losing strength. My right foot was numb by this time. I knew something was wrong, but eight doctors, including three chiropractors, could not identify the problem. Then, by accident, a technician at Mercy Hospital in Iowa City discovered a lesion on my lower lung as he examined a stomach MRI. In alarm, the doctor immediately sent me to a surgeon for a biopsy.

You Have Cancer!

Dr. A. was firm but gentle when he spoke the fateful words, "Your lungs are filled with cancer." He went on to say this particular cancer was inoperable. Of course, I was shocked; we all were.

As a pastor and counselor, I knew the first stage of grief is denial. Well, I was in denial for some days. I couldn't believe I had cancer. Dr. G., who first discovered the abnormality in my lungs from the CAT scan, had quizzed me in a way that should have prepared me for the dire diagnosis.

"Do you smoke?"

"No!"

"Have you ever smoked?"

"No."

"Have you been around a lot of secondhand smoke?"

"No."

"Well, cancer has its own mind. Some people who smoke all their lives don't get it and some people who never smoked do get it. I'm sending you to a cancer specialist."

Following exploratory surgery, the cancer specialist later ameliorated his grim diagnosis to something happier. "You have aggressive lymphoma which has settled in your lungs. This is very unusual." He went on to say that lymphoma is treatable and the survival rate is greater than for lung cancer. But that didn't change the facts: I had Stage 4, inoperable cancer that had already spread to my other lung.

At the time, I wrote a post for my blog at www.bmarkanderson.com: "If need be, I'm ready to die. I have received Jesus Christ as my Savior from the guilt of my sin. According to God's Word, I am secure in His love and forgiveness, and I will be with Him when I die. In the meantime, I will try to beat this thing by the power of God and the prayers of His people. That's my confidence in God and His Word. If I do die, I don't want to die of cancer. I believe if someone is going to die, they should die healthy!"

I remember one poignant statement the biopsy doctor made: "Your life will change. You are headed for some rough days ahead." Little did I know what he meant or what traumas I would soon face.

Your Life Will Change

I knew I needed to let our church in on the recent diagnosis. Just how to tell them I wasn't sure …

My wife, Kari, and some of our children stood on either side of me as I announced to our church that I had cancer. When we sat down, the entire church immediately gathered around us and started ministering to us in faith and prayer. They didn't hesitate one bit. One lady, Sherry, who is herself a cancer survivor, announced with unmitigated faith and passion, "Christ is a big 'C'; cancer is a little 'c'!" There I was, a broken man, and the whole church was standing as one in staunch faith and love.

Who are the majestic ones? "As for the saints who are in the earth, they are the majestic ones in whom is all my delight" (Psalm 16). The church of the Living Water stood by me like an immoveable rock throughout the duration of my chemotherapy treatments. If I didn't know it before (and I did), I know it now—the saints of God, the church, are the majestic ones in all the earth.

My wife and family, all seven of our children, gave me unwavering assistance throughout the trial. They are majestic in my eyes.

My fellow pastors in Muscatine rallied to my benefit. God heard prayers from the pulpits of nearly every church in town. Baptist, Methodist, Vineyard, non-denominational, and so on, they all prayed for me. These are a majestic band of brothers.

"A brother in need is a brother indeed." The aphorism is true. Crisis reveals our true friends. Nor should anyone be surprised that Christian people are salient in the mercy department. Every believer in Jesus Christ has received His mercy. It's only natural that we pass it on.

If the cruel monster called cancer is traumatizing you or someone you know, consider contacting the ministry team at The Church of the Living Water in Muscatine, Iowa. Someone will listen to you and pray with you.

It's common in some quarters to criticize the church in America. Yet when the chips are down, who is the greatest support group anywhere? Unbelievers need to know there is an assembly of "Good Samaritans" ready and willing to help in time of need. Wow, what a tremendous support group! May God strengthen the church in the eyes of the unsaved!

The biopsy doctor made an appointment for me to see Dr. James Feeley, head of the Cancer Care Center in Iowa City, Iowa. Dr. Feeley is one of the most sensitive and compassionate men I've met. He is also a brilliant oncologist. After one look at me, he immediately sent me to the hospital and began chemotherapy. I had no time to consider other options. Nor was I in any condition to consider options. By this time I was failing fast.

Although I didn't know it at the time, I realized later that Dr. Feeley's intervention saved my life.

Only God knows what would have happened if I had known anything at all about alternative therapies. At this point in my life I thought alternative treatments were "hokey" (and a few of them are).

Even in the middle of cancer and side effects, humor breaks out. One of my daughters and I had fun making a list of the "cancer cures" people suggested. Most of these came unsolicited from well-meaning folks who knew nothing about cancer.

The worst idea of all was "drink your own urine." How that was supposed to cure, I never found out. I never tried it, and somehow, even the thought of it left a bad taste in my mouth! Another suggestion was the "carrot diet." Carrots are good for us, of course, and do contain cancer-healing properties. But to limit the diet to carrots turns the skin yellow. Oh, well, I'd rather be yellow than dead.

Or try to cure cancer with the "soda diet." Actually, baking soda can help, but just gulping down mega amounts of baking soda won't cut it. The same with the "hydrogen peroxide treatment."

One of my favorites from friends was the ketogenic diet, which is really a starvation diet. Truthfully, this diet can actually work; it starves cancer cells—and the person who's in the cells too! For me, however, I'm lean to start with, had already lost nearly thirty pounds, and was heading downhill fast. When I looked in the mirror, I thought I was a holocaust survivor. If only the people who suggested this diet could have seen me, they would have never mentioned the ketogenic diet.

Traumatic Treatments

I began a series of six chemotherapy treatments. The first were the worst. As I wrote on my blog at www.bmarkanderson.com:

> I experienced hell. No place on earth is like hell. If we care about anyone, we will do our best to rescue him or her from the ravages of the devil and his place of torment.
>
> Following my first chemotherapy treatment I was reduced to a near vegetable state. I was weak physically, and weaker still in my mind. In a drug-induced stupor I was susceptible to demonic attack. As I tried to sleep that first night, I felt all hell was turned upside down and poured out on me. Hideous, evil thoughts I'd never seen or imagined camped in my mind.
>
> I do deliverance ministry. I know how to combat the devil. But this was different. When I called for the blood of Jesus, the devil himself seemed to appear. I couldn't get free no matter what I tried. What I experienced was the horrendous hatred of the devil toward me and every human being. No words can adequately describe the devil and his hatred. No words can fully prepare a person for the torments of hell. No place on earth is like it. I repeat, if we care about anyone, we will do our best to rescue him or her from the ravages of the devil and his place of torment.
>
> The next night I came armed with the prayers of my oldest son and the elders of the church. Through their prayers I was greatly, although not entirely, protected.
>
> I see now more clearly than ever the need to rescue people from the devil's deception and bring them into heaven. If we care at all about friends, relatives, or co-workers we will tell them about Jesus. No feeling should stop us from giving the good news about salvation from hell to people we care about. I say again, if we love

someone, let's spare nothing in order to tell them about Jesus and lead them to salvation. (See some posts on my blog, "Chicken Evangelism" for simple, empowering ways to lead someone to Christ—it's serious business, but also a lot of fun!)

Hell is neither a picnic nor place to go and party with friends. Learn about Chicken Evangelism—share Christ before you chicken out. If we love 'em, tell 'em about Jesus now!"

Cured?

After six chemotherapy treatments, things looked good. I was feeling better, and tests showed no sign of the cancerous tumors in my lungs. The doctor and the head nurse used the word "cure." I sent out a health update to all my supporters announcing the good news. "Tests show I am cancer-free," I reported. I went about my business and began to gain strength.

Shock!

After a month I returned for the 30-day checkup. The results came with a jolt—something for which I was not prepared. I had expected the test to confirm my good health, but instead the MRI showed a tennis-ball-sized tumor in my lung.

A surgical biopsy confirmed the diagnosis: cancer had returned with a vengeance! Dr. A., the physician who performed the biopsy, had already made an appointment for me to have a portion of my lung surgically removed. (He made the appointment without consulting me!) He explained this procedure was major surgery. Part of my rib cage would have to be cut out. He also said I needed chemotherapy immediately, but with the surgery, there would be a six-week recovery period before chemotherapy could resume.

The doctor gravely announced, "If you take chemotherapy treatments, you have a 10 percent chance of survival." I didn't like the odds …

What were we to do? By this time we had learned a few things regarding alternative treatments. The Cancer Tutor website was the beginning of my instruction. I strongly desired to avoid chemotherapy, if possible. I told the doctor I wanted to delay decisions regarding surgery and chemo in order to develop a treatment strategy.

Of course, I turned to God. One of the first Scriptures that "registered" with me was "Christ redeemed us from the curse of the Law, having become a curse for us—for it is written, 'Cursed is everyone who hangs on a tree'" (Galatians 3:13). This truth gripped me as I meditated on it. I knew Christ had redeemed me from the curse of the Law, which is sickness. Healing seemed at hand.

I began some awful-tasting and aggressive alternative treatments using the little knowledge we had accrued by that time.

But it was too late. My left lung started bleeding profusely, so profusely that I was not able to lie on my back long enough to take another MRI. During one of the tests, my blood began to spurt out through my mouth. The attendants hustled me off the MRI machine and out of the room in a flash!

The medical establishment is superb in two areas. Doctors and laboratories are great about diagnosis (although I admit they discovered the original cancer plaguing my body only with delay and difficulty). Further, the crown jewel of modern medicine is emergency intervention. Thankfully, I received the best of intervention at the most critical time. Dr. Feeley and the best of modern medicine were instrumental in saving my life a second time.

I had no choice but to undergo more chemo treatments. Fortunately, chemo went better this second round of eight treatments. I didn't experience hell like before. Nor did I lose my hair.

Hope from God's Word

My wife's cousin Greta mailed us a small folder of healing Scriptures that Joyce Meyer compiled. Those Scriptures comforted me and built my faith. Day after day, too weak to walk without help, that little folder of healing Scriptures became a daily source of strength. I can't express how much this little brochure meant to me. Daily confession and meditation on God's word proved life-giving. Those Scriptures and even the format became the basis for this current book.

While meditating on Isaiah 55:11, a liberating truth dawned on me. Take a look at this marvelous portion of Scripture:

> For as the rain and the snow come down from heaven, and do not return there without watering the earth and making it bear and sprout, and furnishing seed to the sower and bread to the eater; so will My word be which goes forth from My mouth; It will not

return to Me empty, without accomplishing what I desire, and without succeeding in the matter for which I sent it.

I realized every word of God has a specific purpose. Each word will accomplish what it was sent to do. The word contains the power to produce what it says. Just as when God said, "Let there be light" and there was light, healing Scriptures contain the capacity to produce healing. Just as raindrops activate the natural processes of the soil, so healing words activate the natural healing processes of the body.

"Wow!" I thought, "I can't lose. I may never be sick again!" I knew God was healing me. Though I wrestled with doubts sometimes, I expected complete healing from lymphoma would come either suddenly or gradually.

Hope from God's Spirit

As I reflect back, I'm amazed at God's faithfulness to encourage me. My journal entries frequently report dreams or "waking thoughts" signifying God's healing. On April 16, 2013, I was wearing braces on both legs and walking with a cane. Yet that night I awoke with a dream that I had forgotten to take my cane. I was walking fast (almost running) and was carrying out the garbage! Talk about a faith-builder!

On May 20, 2013 God impressed me with these words regarding healing: "Don't give up!" The story from Luke 18 about the widow woman who never gave up accompanied that message.

On May 31, 2013 I wrote this entry in my journal. "Dream! I was playing basketball with young boys. I could jump and shoot and play! PTL!"

In July of 2013 my wife Kari, who is very sensitive to the Holy Spirit, heard these words: "I will heal your husband soon."

On July 26, 2013 God again spoke to Kari: "Your husband IS healed. You will see." This was accompanied with a vision of a steady, gradual healing.

From the beginning, Kari and I bathed my condition with fervent prayer and meditation on healing Scriptures. Oftentimes I felt the surge of faith in God for healing. Several times I sensed God's immediate healing power in my body.

Once I walked into an Aglow meeting. The women stopped everything and prayed for me. I walked away sensing, "I'm healed by the power of God." The sensation was noteworthy. Praise God!

Individuals and churches in more than one country prayed for me for which I am eternally grateful. Because of those prayers and the mercy of God, I am alive today. Miraculously, it never once crossed my mind during those days that I might die from cancer.

But still the symptoms of chest pain and numbness in my feet persisted.

The Truth Begins to Dawn: 5-Year Survival Percentage Rates

Kari and I slowly began to realize the life-changing truth: Standard medical intervention and treatment rarely cure cancer. Multiple sources report the cancer cure rate with chemotherapy is only about 2 or 3 percent!

One of the best large-scale studies on the effectiveness of chemotherapy treatments—the main weapon in the cancer war—was published in 2004. This study was not conducted by some bitter scientist, but by two highly respected oncologists from Australia. They simply looked at the results of every randomized, controlled clinical trial performed in the United States between 1990 and 2004 which reported a statistically significant increase in five-year survival due to chemotherapy. That is, they looked at the number of cancer patients who survived more than five years following diagnosis and treatment. Here are the results:

Bladder	0.0%
Kidney	0.0%
Melanoma	0.0%
Multiple Myeloma	0.0%
Pancreas	0.0%
Prostate	0.0%
Soft-tissue sarcoma	0.0%
Unknown primary site	0.0%
Uterus	0.0%
Stomach	0.7%
Colon	1.0%
Breast	1.4%
Head and neck	1.7%
Lung	2.0%
Rectum	3.4%
Brain	3.7%
Esophagus	4.9%
Ovary	8.9%

Non-Hodgkin's lymphoma	10.5%
Cervix	12.0%
Testis	37.7%
Hodgkin's disease	40.3%
Overall 5-Year Survival Rate	**2.1%**[1]

Hope Beyond Chemotherapy

After examining chemo cure rates and scouring various treatment options, my wife and I arrived at some startling conclusions. We realized that if I were going to survive, we must look beyond chemotherapy and conventional medicine.

Yes, chemotherapy had done its job: it had killed cysts and millions of deadly cancer cells. It had given me the gift of time to educate myself and take responsibility for my healing. Tests revealed no noticeable tumors in my lung. Relieved, we began to pray for a maintenance program to keep cancer away.

Our son Andrew gave us a copy of Bill Henderson's *How to Cure Almost Any Cancer at Home for $5.15 a Day*. This book became an answer to our prayers. When Henderson's wife suffered and eventually died through cancer treatments, he decided there must be a better way. Thorough investigation with oncologists, researchers, and cancer patients led him to discover gentle and inexpensive cancer treatments that work. He explains and simplifies complex issues in a way most of us can understand.

Bill Henderson became our chief "cancer coach." More accurately, he became our "health mentor." For the main part, I follow Henderson's protocol today.

Mysteries

What caused cancer in my body? I don't know. I have consulted with nine doctors; none can say what caused cancer in my body. I understand that innumerable cancer cells reside in the body of every healthy person. Only when the immune system becomes overwhelmed does cancer become a problem. Toxins, stress, and other causes can overpower God's normal plan for healing—the immune system.

---

[1] Clinical Oncology (2004) 16:549e560; doi 10.1016/j.clon.2004.06.07

When did I first get cancer? I don't know that either. Apparently, cancer had been growing for some time in my body before diagnosis.

When was I healed of lymphoma? This is yet another mystery. Once, a man named Jerry Hopper, a veteran minister who has experienced a variety of dramatic acts of God, prayed for me. Perhaps God touched me at that time. Pastor Hopper later confided that in all his years of ministry, he had never felt such a powerful anointing as that time he laid his hands on me for healing.

It's safest to say that many factors, both natural and spiritual, contributed to my healing.

The last thing I want is the return of cancer. Between Thanksgiving and Christmas in 2011 the first symptoms leading to a cancer diagnosis appeared. Today I am strong, working full time from before dawn until late at night doing what God is calling me to do. For recreation and exercise, I chop wood, climb ladders, lift weights (beginner and intermediate level), and help on our farm.

When I wrote *Answer for Cancer: 9 Keys* I thought it could help other people. As I look back, I recognize I was writing it for me! By daily writing and mulling over the Scriptures, truth came into my innermost being. From my spirit, life-giving truth "leaked out" into every cell of my body. I'm alive and well today because of the power of God's word imprinted upon my body.

Epigenetics refers to external modifications to DNA that turn genes "on" or "off." While these modifications do not change the DNA sequence, they impact the health and behavior of every organism, including humans. Meditation is one example of an external modification that powerfully affects human health.

The study of epigenetics helped me understand Jesus' words in Mark 11:22-24:

> And Jesus answered saying to them, "Have faith in God. Truly, I say to you, whoever says to this mountain, 'Be taken up and cast into the sea,' and does not doubt in his heart, but believes that what he says is going to happen, it will be granted him. Therefore I say to you, all things for which you pray and ask, believe that you have received them, and they will be granted you."

Through meditation and confession of God's word, I received His word. His life-giving energy affected every cell and organism in my body.

I thank God I'm alive. Together with Kari, I look forward to the next thirty or more years of life on earth. We have plans, hopes, and dreams. As God allows, we will serve His church, write, travel, develop the farm, increase our businesses, thrive, and prosper.

> Now to Him who is able to do far more abundantly beyond all that we ask or think, according to the power that works within us, to Him be the glory in the church and in Christ Jesus to all generations forever and ever. Amen (Ephesians 3:20-21).

Almost every organization has someone suffering from cancer. I can bring hope and encouragement to your college, church, club, or group. Contact me to speak by coming to BMarkAnderson.com and filling in the contact form. When people get the life-saving information in this book, they can thrive!

All healing is from God. As I look back, I realize God healed me through a process of nine natural and spiritual actions which I consider essential. Some actions only God could do, some were my responsibility; both were essential. I detail those actions in Part Two and Part Three of ***Answer for Cancer: 9 Keys.***

There is hope for all!

Part Two

Cancer is a Formidable Foe: Nine Natural and Spiritual Keys for Prevention and Cure

Gather all the forces of heaven and nature to combat this killer disease. As I learned about cancer, I developed a strategy with nine keys. Some are natural, some spiritual. Why nine? Because cancer is a multifaceted monster with far-reaching tentacles.

These nine (or at least most of them) must be done simultaneously. It's not enough to build your immune system, but not deal with diet. It's not enough to change your diet, but not detoxify. It's not enough to detoxify without alkalizing. It's not enough to deal with the natural without facing the emotional and spiritual issues.

An internationally recognized prophetic minister died from a reoccurrence of cancer on February 15, 2015. This man was a hero to me and many others. At a meeting in St. Paul, Minnesota, he picked me out of a crowd and spoke over me things that only God and I knew. He prophesied that I would write and travel, the very things I was privately praying about. He was a giant of faith who had earlier experienced a miraculous recovery from cancer surgery. Yet he died at a relatively young age. I am not privy to all the facts, yet none of the vast information from him or about him gave any indication that he was addressing natural issues such as the keys in this book.

These nine components are tried and true and have become a natural part of my life. Each is valuable even for healthy people who do not have cancer or any other disease. These nine keys are so potent they may help prevent disease from ever occurring. And I repeat, these nine must be done simultaneously.

Alternative doctors are using a variety of treatments to cure cancer. Please see the Additional Resources at the back of this book for further information. I don't wish to imply the resources in this book are the only way. Yet they have worked for me and thousands of others. Do your research and decide what is best for you. Cancer is not a death sentence!

Chapter 1

First Key: Get a Coach

Or better yet, get several coaches. There's no way the doctor can break the news gently. Invariably, the dire diagnosis comes as a shock. When the physician reports, "You've got cancer!" most of us are hit with a whirlwind of emotions: "Are you sure?" "Could the tests be wrong?" "Do we need more tests?" What about a second opinion?" "What's next?" "What did I do wrong?" "Why?" and on and on. The questions never end.

First, the diagnosis hits with locomotive force. Then denial, anger, confusion, and grief follow like cars on a freight train. They did for me. Sometimes there are no apparent answers. That's why I have written *Answer for Cancer: 9 Keys*.

Your best shot is to learn about cancer, get a coach, and take personal responsibility for your own health.

A question often asked of medical doctors, especially oncologists, is "What would you do if you were diagnosed with cancer?" Cancer survivors are also asked, "I've been diagnosed with cancer. What do you recommend I do?"

My answer is prayerfully search out a health coach. This answer may surprise you. I don't hear it from others, yet I can't say it loudly enough: Get a coach. Even if you don't have cancer now, get a health coach!

I didn't say, "Find a doctor." I said, "Find a health coach." Your doctor can help with diagnosis, emergency treatment, and medication, but is probably not your best health coach. Doctors are trained to diagnose and treat symptoms, not cure cancer. Medical schools offer little or no training in nutrition, which is vital for healing cancer.

Has your doctor ever talked with you about your diet? How much time has your doctor spent with you discussing nutrition? Has your doctor ever mentioned detoxification to you? Diet and detox are both highly significant health issues in our highly toxic environment. Both are outside the realm of the training and expertise of the medical profession.

In stating these facts, I don't intend to denigrate medical doctors or the medical profession in the least. On the contrary, let's face reality. Doctors are specialists; generally they have no expertise outside the realm of their credentials. My own oncologist, Dr. James Feeley of the Cancer Care Center in Iowa City, is a splendid man and exceptionally competent oncologist. He is a specialist. He knows chemotherapy and could not be more qualified in what he does. However, he is not a health coach to help navigate life or health issues outside the realms of cancer and chemotherapy.

Why is a health mentor a matter of critical import? Because of the complexity of environmental toxicities in the world today. Add to that the uniqueness and complexity of each human body. These issues are nearly unfathomable and largely outside the scope of our current educational and medical systems.

We are, however, responsible for our own health and health decisions. Personal responsibility in this most important area—our own health—is often lacking. I, for one, took my health for granted until I got cancer.

Why locate a health coach? Look around. World-class athletes choose a mentor (or mentors) to shave a few seconds off their time in search of Olympic gold. Successful business entrepreneurs select a mentor to guide them through the complexities of a profitable business. Those breaking into financial services do the same. Farmers pay mega bucks for consultants and crop scouts to get the highest yields. Christians commit themselves to churches and pastors for life guidance and spiritual tutelage. How many of us locate a coach to prevent disease and guide us toward optimum health?

Several mentors may be helpful. The Bible says, "For by wise guidance you will wage war, and in abundance of counselors there is victory" (Proverbs 24:6). No one will ever know all there is to learn about cancer. However, some doctors and researchers with open minds have been curing cancer for decades. Some have proven records of accomplishment and know what has worked to help hundreds or thousands to overcome this devastating disease.

When I got my cancer diagnosis, I had no knowledge, no idea, no money, and no silver bullets to understand or battle cancer. I do now.

My best source of early information became Webster Kerr, former webmaster at CancerTutor.com and vice president of the Independent Cancer Research Foundation. Although a Wikipedia article labels him a quack, I disagree. I found Webster to be an honest and informed researcher. His website and recommendations of other advisors with whom I have personal experience were instrumental to my own recovery from cancer. Anyone who reads the home page at CancerTutor.com will learn more about cancer and the pharmaceutical industry than many will learn in a lifetime.

A coach can help us find the cause of our cancer. How can we overcome this formidable foe if we don't know the cause? Numerous factors may contribute to the cause, including but not limited to: parasites, fungi, viruses, bacteria, and stress. Don't forget about pesticides, herbicides, and household chemicals.

Together with my wife, we chose Bill Henderson as a coach. I first heard about him from Webster Kerr on the above-mentioned site. In *Cancer-Free: Your Guide to Gentle, Non-Toxic Healing*, Henderson and co-author Carlos M. Garcia, MD lay out three basic causes of most cancers, which they say must be addressed and corrected in order for healing to occur:

1. Stress: Whether from an event like the sudden loss of a family member, or extended emotional stress, like that caused by a bitter divorce, stress is a triggering factor for many diseases.

2. Dental toxins: Root canals, cavitation, and metal fillings suppress the immune system and allow cancer, an opportunistic condition, to grow.

3. What we put in our mouths: Cigarettes and alcohol trigger cancer growth, but so do some cooked and packaged foods, which have no enzymes and few nutrients and can't be adequately digested.

Some of these factors are easily overlooked by the uninitiated (which includes most of us). That's why we need a coach or mentor to guide us in the cancer war. The guide can be a person, a book, a website, or a combination of all these. Just don't try to go the distance alone!

Another health guide for me is Starla Weichman of Be Healthy Naturally. What this company can do by analyzing hair, nail, urine, and saliva samples amazes me. I give credit to Starla for discovering and treating two types of Lyme's Disease in me, which can cause cancer. Starla Weichman's company also determined I had parasites and candida overload, both of which can cause cancer.

In choosing a coach, I suggest examining at least five areas.

1. Is he or she Biblical? There's a lot of advice that sounds good, but just doesn't agree with the New Testament. This is my area of expertise so I've had to discard much advice that seemed good at first but ended up to be pure humanism.

Think about this for a moment. The Bible warns about *"men who forbid marriage and advocate abstaining from foods which God has created to be gratefully shared in by those who believe and know the truth. For everything created by God is good, and nothing is to be rejected if it is received with gratitude; for it is sanctified by means of the word of God and prayer"* (1 Timothy 4:3-5).

Why do some counselors exclude all dairy and meat? Often, more than one coach is needed in order to get well-rounded information.

2. What's he selling? I'm not opposed to anyone developing a product and making a profit from it. However, we should investigate, run reviews, and do our own due diligence on anything that is going into our minds and bodies.

3. What kind of a record of accomplishment does he have? How long has he been doing this? Again, a bit of investigation is worth the time. Our life could depend on it. Is he actually curing cancer, or is he merely treating symptoms? How do you know? What are others saying about him?

4. How available is he or she? Does he have a website for current information? Books? Does he answer email? Can you reach him via telephone or in person? A coach need not be someone you talk with personally, but the more available, the better.

5. Does he understand and appreciate the difference between grassfed and conventional meat and milk? Some well-qualified mentors prohibit meat and dairy products because they have not distinguished between grassfed products and conventional meat or dairy. There's more about this in Chapter 8, "Diet, Nutrition, and Cooking."

Having stated the importance of due diligence in choosing a cancer coach, please realize you may not agree with an expert in every area. Nevertheless, we can all learn from veteran counselors. The point is this: find a mentor or mentors you respect and don't try to navigate the troubled waters alone.

While you're researching and selecting a cancer coach, there's something else almost universally overlooked that is vitally important. Taking this action daily continues to grow in significance for me. It's the subject of the next chapter and I believe it's a primary reason I am healed today.

Chapter 2

Second Key: See You Later, Meditator

Plenty of scientifically accredited research shows those who meditate live longer and are healed faster than those who don't. To put it bluntly, if you want to continue living a good life on planet earth, learn to meditate on God's word.

At first glance by logical, intelligent people, it seems counter-intuitive that something so simple as meditation could have any effect whatever on health. The scientific evidence, however, strongly supports the fact that meditation enhances healing and health.

Emma Seppälä, PhD, is Associate Director of the Center for Compassion and Altruism Research and Education at Stanford University. She obtained her BA from Yale, her MA from Columbia University and her PhD in psychology from Stanford University. She lists multiple positive outcomes of meditation.[2]

Meditation decreases pain. It decreases inflammation at the cellular level. Meditation boosts our immune system. Even short mindfulness meditation sessions boost memory and creativity.

Meditation decreases stress and anxiety, both of which contribute to sickness and disease, including cancer. Meditation contributes to a positive mental outlook and emotional well-being. Meditation decreases depression. All of the above assist in the fight to overcome cancer.

Here's an example of a benefit of Christian meditation. While researching and meditating on healing Scriptures, I discovered that God takes pleasure in healing people! While confessing healing Scriptures I often feel

---

[2] https://www.psychologytoday.com/blog/feeling-it/201309/20-scientific-reasons-start-meditating-today (last accessed June 4, 2015).

God's pleasure and sense His healing presence. What a wonderful sensation! There's more about this in Part Three.

Meditation connects a person with God's heart, and that's the key. Jesus can be the Sole Solution, or at the very least, a source of the solution to one of life's most disturbing diseases—cancer. By spending time in His presence, He can direct you to the best clinic, doctor, or treatment for your particular situation. He did for me.

Many forms of meditation can become health intensifiers. I concentrate on meditation on God and His word because it's as old as Moses and is backed by promises of health and longevity by God Himself. A critical action to keep a cancer sufferer alive is *meditate on God and His word*.

Meditation goes beyond prayer and reading the Bible. Believers often shoot "arrow" prayers to the heavens. Or sometimes we pray memorized prayers. Either can be positive and meaningful. Hopefully, all who read this are already committing some time on a regular basis for Bible reading or study. However, none of this is the same as meditation. Meditation includes, yet involves more than "quality time with God."

Meditation is like an intravenous feeding where God's substance drips into our veins and fills us with the life and character of God Himself. Meditation is the gentle art of mulling over and "digesting" God's word.

Allowing God's word to float through my mind is helping me comprehend the nature of God Himself. Through meditation, truth is seeping into me. I'm learning that healing is about God and not about me. Healing and miracles are the very nature of God. Fish swim, eagles soar, water wets, God heals. It's all natural. It's reality. It's the way things are. Healing is something God does and the manner and timing are up to Him. Meditation is God's method to open our eyes. It's one of God's chosen and gentle means to bring reality.

Christian meditation on God's word involves taking time, quieting the soul with mental, emotional, and spiritual focus. Christian meditation can produce such benefits as inner peace, stress reduction, and release of tension, frustration, and anxiety. It can and does yield improved health and well-being, better memory, and clearer focus on life's priorities.

Christian meditation is not cessation of thought; rather, it is concentration on God and His word with the goal of spiritual, emotional, and mental union with Christ Jesus. As God pours Himself into our human spirit, His Holy Spirit transforms us in every realm of life, including the physical. That's how healing takes place. God first feeds our spirit, and then His transforming life goes into our body and mind.

Christian meditation is generally verbal. The Hebrew word *hagah* can be translated meditate, murmur, mutter, utter, muse, speak, or even growl (like a lion over its prey). It's used of the gentle sounds of the cooing of a dove. Christian meditation often involves the half-aloud reading and re-reading of God's word.

Take Deuteronomy 7:15 as an example:

And the LORD will remove from you all sickness … The Lord WILL remove from you all sickness. The Lord will REMOVE from you all sickness. The Lord will remove FROM you all sickness. The Lord will remove from YOU all sickness. The Lord will remove from you ALL sickness. The Lord will remove from you all SICKNESS.

You get the picture. By mulling over each word, truth is planted and faith is born.

Yes, I know that yoga and other forms of meditation can be calming for body and mind, but why not go for the best and most powerful? God's word is perhaps the most dynamic source of peace and strength on planet Earth.

What does this have to do with healing? By now, science and the medical establishment are well aware of the healing ability of meditation. As noted in the section regarding community support (Chapter 3), even Medicare pays people who meditate under certain conditions!

Meditation is not as easy as we might think. If it were, we'd do more of it.

I have discovered a major problem regarding meditation, or more precisely, the lack of it. Many people believe in meditation, but fail to practice it. Many know about it and have experienced its benefits, yet have gotten sporadic or abandoned the practice altogether.

This is true in my own life. When I was desperate for healing from cancer and my life was hanging in the balance, I spent more time meditating on healing Scriptures. This was due to the fact that I was largely incapacitated—I couldn't do much else. Now I'm up and around, feeling pressure to accomplish my goals and help other people. Consequently, I meditate less.

Here's another problem. I tend to want to rush through a meditation session to get on with "more important" things. It's a discipline to take a "Sabbath time" to rest, release, and meditate. Yet, rest must be a crucial part of meditation. If we don't quiet ourselves, how can we call it meditation? For God's sake, let's quiet down!

Authors have published volumes pertaining to diet and other matters of natural health. As I peruse the literature regarding cancer and healing of other diseases, one of the most neglected aspects is the spiritual dimension. That's one of the reasons I have invested time in this book.

What action can you take to keep yourself alive? Faith-building confession and meditation on God's word, repentance of any known sin, and forgiveness are vital for health. Our loving God sent His Son to earth and the cross for our forgiveness and healing. While spiritual healing via meditation on God's word is the central focus of this book, neglect of natural aspects of health may prove fatal.

People don't need to die from cancer. Cancer is not a death sentence, no matter what someone says. Natural and spiritual treatments are available and working. Many of these treatments are free, gentle, simple, inexpensive, and can be accomplished at home.

For emphasis, I repeat: God's power for faith and healing came on me as I mused over His word. Meditation on God and His word became major factors in my healing. If you find meditation on healing Scriptures from the Bible is helping you, pass the truth on to someone you know. Give them a copy of *Answer for Cancer: 9 Keys* and let them know the power.

The cancer patient needs every weapon he can get in his arsenal. Don't neglect the most powerful: meditation on God and His word.

While the value of meditation in our busy world is often overlooked and undervalued, here's another wonder: scientific research verifies the role of love and group support for those seeking healing.

Chapter 3

Third Key: Love Can Save Your Life!

We're talking here about good, old-fashioned love and support. Few cancer sufferers survive and thrive without some type of support group. Emotional and spiritual support can come from either formal or informal groups, or both.

For me, it's my family and church.

The importance of a support group is something we know intuitively, yet has been overlooked by the scientific community in past years. But no more.

On January 1, 2010 Medicare began covering people who qualify under the program of lifestyle change developed by Dr. Dean Ornish. One of the four parts of his program involves a support group. His research demonstrates that people who join or are part of a support group recover more rapidly from disease. He's not talking about something difficult or expensive. He's simply referring to good, old-fashioned love and encouragement from a surrounding cadre of caring people.

Dean Ornish, MD, is the founder and president of the non-profit Preventive Medicine Research Institute and is Clinical Professor of Medicine at the University of California, San Francisco. Dr. Ornish has directed clinical research demonstrating that comprehensive lifestyle changes may begin to reverse even severe coronary heart disease, without drugs or surgery.

He directed the first randomized controlled trial demonstrating that comprehensive lifestyle changes may slow, stop or reverse the progression of early-stage prostate cancer. His current research showed that comprehensive lifestyle changes affect gene expression, "turning on" disease-preventing genes and "turning off" genes that promote cancer and heart disease.[3]

Dr. Tony Jimenez, MD, founder of the Hope 4 Cancer Institute asserts, "A negative thought can kill you faster than a bad germ." A cadre of positive, encouraging friends who speak life-giving words contribute to healing. Emotional and spiritual support need not come only from organized groups. As indicated above, informal groups such as families and communities often bolster one's ability to sustain a healthful lifestyle. Few people are able to go it alone. We all need reinforcement from surrounding friends, relatives, and allies to maintain healthful choices.

From where does your support for a healthy lifestyle come? If you have strong encouragement regarding diet, exercise, and the other actions in this book, great! If not, find your group! Love and support are keystones to keep you alive.

What about the miracles of modern medicine? Why can't I just take my pills and get well?

---

[3] http://www.pmri.org/dean_ornish.html (last accessed January 29, 2015).

Chapter 4

Fourth Key: Modern Medicine—Mixture of Miracle and Murder

The crown jewels of modern medicine are diagnosis and emergency intervention. I needed both to save my life. Without doctors, medicines, hospitals, diagnostic tools, and various medical equipment, I most likely would not be alive today. I thank God for all the money, research, time, and expertise that have gone into the development and practice of modern medicine.

When the doctor says, "You've got cancer!" most people quickly rely on the best of modern medicine. That included me. I knew nothing of alternative treatments that were actually curing cancer and had been doing so for decades, possibly millennia. Others, having had negative experiences or expecting too much from doctors and medicine, speak disparagingly of conventional medicine. These tend to downplay or deny the nearly supernatural results of modern medical procedures. Let not anyone who wears prescription eyeglasses fall into this trap!

We should all marvel at what modern medicine can do. The author is a cancer survivor who discovered his own brain cancer on his own brain resonance equipment. This excerpt from *Anti Cancer: A New Way of Life* by David Sesravan-Schreiber, MD, PhD says it well as he writes of a myocardial infarction (heart attack):

> A patient arrives in the emergency room on the point of death—pale, suffocating with crushing pain in her chest. The medical team, guided by years of cutting-edge research on tens of thousands of patients, knows exactly what to do: in a few minutes, oxygen is flowing through nasal prongs; nitroglycerin is dilating her veins; a beta-blocker is slowing down her heart rate; a dose of aspirin is

preventing the creation of additional clots; and morphine is relieving her pain. In less than ten minutes, this woman's life has been saved. She breathes normally, she speaks to her family, and she even smiles. This is the miracle of medicine in what it has most spectacularly and most admirably to offer.[4]

At the same time, medicine in its current state can be an accomplice to murder. I don't suggest this lightly. Nor do I want to say it. At least two decades ago I read multiple reports and refused to believe them. By now, however, the cat is out of the bag. The FDA and the AMA have suppressed legitimate cures for cancer and persecuted doctors who are successfully treating cancer patients. Any google search for "FDA cancer cure cover-up" will show numerous articles regarding this sad circumstance. Books by reliable authors detail the same information and expose the FDA, some hospitals, the pharmaceutical industry, and the AMA.

To withhold life-saving information and to suppress legitimate cures while cancer sufferers die is serving as an accomplice to murder. While modern medicine can and does produce miraculous results, the entire health care industry needs its own physician.

Here's another eye-opening statistic. The overall contribution of curative and adjuvant cytotoxic chemotherapy to 5-year survival in adults was estimated to be 2.3% in Australia and 2.1% in the USA.[5]

From Webster Kerr at CancerTutor.com we find the following excerpt:

[T]he 5-year cure rate [for cancer] in America is 2.1%. In other words, in five years after diagnosis, 97.9% of the cancer patients treated with traditional cancer treatments, meaning those who trust the media and pharmaceutical industry, are dead.

So what are the cancer treatments with 90% cure rates that the media is hiding? I will give you one quick example.

The late Dr. William D. Kelley, a dentist turned cancer researcher, treated over 33,000 cancer patients. Among those who went to him first, his 5-year cure rate was 90%.

Why hasn't the media glorified Dr. Kelley? The reason is that Dr. Kelley used products that cannot be patented.

---

[4] *Anti Cancer: A New Way of Life* (2008, Viking Press).
[5] http://www.burtongoldberg.com/home/burtongoldberg/contribution-of-chemotherapy-to-five-year-survival-rate-morgan.pdf (last accessed May 19, 2015).

It is patents that create massive profits for the media and the pharmaceutical industry and the medical industry!! Because Dr. Kelley did not use patented drugs, the media doesn't talk about him and no one in the medical industry is using his safe, gentle and highly effective protocol (with one exception in New York – the clinic of Dr. Nicholas Gonzalez).

So what did Dr. Kelley use? He used treatments designed by God. The problem is that orthodox medicine refuses to use treatments that cannot be patented! That, in a nutshell, is the difference between orthodox medicine and natural medicine! Orthodox medicine uses highly profitable treatments and we use safe, gentle, and highly effective treatments.[6]

Healthcare suffers crises today. Preventable medical errors in hospitals are the third leading cause of death in the United States. Only heart disease and cancer kill more Americans.[7]

There's plenty of room to pass the blame around. My purpose is not to castigate doctors, hospitals, pharmaceutical companies, the medical profession, government agencies, insurance companies, or even the media. Much of the responsibility for problems in the healthcare industry can be traced to consumers—in other words, you and me.

We the people, like drug-induced teenagers, have failed to take responsibility for our own health. (I, for one, took good health for granted.) Then, when a problem ensues, we expect the doctor to solve it and solve it quickly. We have idolized doctors to the point we consider them little gods. We have given physicians a place they cannot and should not be expected to fill. This attitude is prevalent today. It's simpler to take a pill than to change a life.

My doctor has done everything in his power and within the realm of his expertise to save my life. Mercy Hospital in Iowa City lived up to their name marvelously. A charitable arm of the institution even paid for a portion of my expenses! The Genentech Company (the manufacturer of the chemo drug Rituxan) also paid for a portion of our drug expenses. We came through the chemotherapy treatments debt free without health insurance!

---

[6] http://www.cancertutor.com (last accessed May 19, 2015).
[7] http://www.sanders.senate.gov/newsroom/press-releases/medical-mistakes-are-3rd-leading-cause-of-death-in-us (last accessed October 7, 2015).

Let's give credit where credit is due. The medical complex in America is one of the great achievements of modern times—killing cancer, saving lives, and relieving the suffering from myriad diseases. At the same time, let's be wise. Physicians are human. Each person must take responsibility for his or her own health.

The war against cancer is fraught with surprises. The next chapter contains information that has boggled the minds of some of the world's most intelligent doctors and oncologists. In fact, it's so surprising, many refuse to believe it. Yet it's a major factor in my own healing experience. I practice it every day.

Chapter 5

Fifth Key: Oxygenation—We "Otto" Know by Now

> *Cancer cells react to oxygenation the way a vampire would react to broad daylight. They hate oxygen.*
>
> —Bill Henderson, cancer coach

Dr. Otto Warburg, awarded the Nobel Prize for Medicine in 1931, first postulated his cancer theory in 1924. He discovered a cancer and oxygen connection that showed promise as a cancer cure.

Further research into Warburg's theory showed that when oxygen levels were turned down, cells began to produce energy anaerobically. They ultimately became cancerous when levels went low enough. It took a reduction of 35% in oxygen levels for this to happen.

J. B. Kizer, a biochemist and physicist at Gungnir Research in Portsmouth, Ohio explains

> Since Warburg's discovery, this difference in respiration has remained the most fundamental (and some say, only) physiological difference consistently found between normal and cancer cells. Using cell culture studies, I decided to examine the differential responses of normal and cancer cells to changes in the oxygen environment....
>
> The results that I found were rather remarkable. I found that ... High 02 [oxygen] tensions were lethal to cancer tissue, 95 percent being very toxic, whereas in general, normal tissues were not harmed by high oxygen tensions. It does seem to demonstrate the possibility that if the 02 [oxygen] tensions in cancer tissues can be

elevated, then the cancer tissue may be able to be killed selectively, as it seems that the cancer cells are incapable of handling the 02 [oxygen] in a high 02 [oxygen] environment.[8]

Ma Lan, MD and Joel Wallach, DVD, point out that one type of white blood cells kills cancer by injecting oxygen into cancerous cells. Think about that. One method our natural immune system uses to kill cancer—it shoots oxygen into the cell!

It's not easy to get additional oxygen into cells. Most approaches don't work well. Breathing oxygen is still limited by the amount of hemoglobin available. I also understand acidic pH levels limit the amount of oxygen that can enter inside our cells. Liquid oxygen supplements release oxygen into the blood, but are unable to deliver oxygen into the cells.[9]

In short, many foods and activities can increase oxygen levels in our blood. Some ways to increase general levels of oxygen in the blood are seen below. All are healthful, but what's really needed is a way to get mega amounts of oxygen to permeate the cell walls and into the interior of the cell itself. A delivery mechanism is needed to transport oxygen into cells.

Enter center stage: Dr. Johanna Budwig, an esteemed cancer research scientist, biochemist and physicist in Germany. In 1951, Dr. Budwig discovered an effective transport system that is so simple that many great minds have stumbled over it. She blended cottage cheese with flaxseed oil at a high speed.

The Budwig protocol is one of the most widely used cancer treatments in the world today. Cancer patients have used her lifesaving protocol for over 60 years. It's practiced in Europe for a wide variety of diseases including heart disease, Type 2 diabetes, arthritis, inflammatory diseases, and many others.

Dr. Budwig claimed a success rate with many types of cancers as high as 90%, but due to the current Western style diet and the ever increasing accumulations of toxins, the cure rate may not be as high as several decades ago.

Following World War II, Dr. Budwig developed her "oil protein" diet in order to combat various types of cancer. She recognized that cancer cells

---

[8] http://www.drstallone.com/cancer_article4.htm (last accessed November 18, 2015).
[9] (http://www.cancerfightingstrategies.com/oxygen-and-cancer.html#sthash.8abDPL8g.dpuf (last accessed May 15, 2015).

are anaerobic, meaning they thrive in an environment with low oxygen, and that the metabolism of cancer cells required sugar.

Dr. Budwig recognized that the denatured foods that the majority of people were consuming did not have many of the necessary enzymes and healthy oils for optimal cellular respiration. Many of the modern-day foods had "manufactured fats" now known as hydrogenated fats and trans fats. She connected the dots and realized that in order for healthy cells to process oxygen as fuel they needed specific enzymes from healthy fats.

After much experimentation, she discovered that when she combined sulfur-rich proteins like cottage cheese with flax seed oil (which is a highly unsaturated fatty acid), the healthy unsaturated fatty acids bonded molecularly with the proteins. This made the flaxseed oil water-soluble, allowing it to be absorbed effortlessly through the cell membrane. This instant flood of vital nutrients and enzymes into the cell restored the cell to a healthy aerobic state. Simply put, she recognized that this formula forced oxygen into cancer cells, returning them to a healthy normal state. It also infused healthy cells with mega amounts of oxygen. When healthy cells are flooded with oxygen, they produce more energy and we just plain "feel better."

Let's explain the process in a slightly different way. Oils are not water-soluble. Our bodies, which are composed of about 75% water, simply cannot completely or readily absorb oils. Dr. Budwig developed a process to get the omega-3 fatty acid (the oil) across the cell membrane and into the cells. The flaxseed oil's lipids bind to the rich protein molecules of the cottage cheese. Through a chemical change, the oil then becomes water-soluble and thereby readily absorbed by the cells. The omega-3 in the flaxseed oil works like a magnet on the cell membrane. This attracts oxygen to the cell and also allows the oxygen to enter inside the cell.

OK, few of us fully understand the chemistry involved. And we don't need to. The discovery took years of meticulous research and experimentation coupled with sheer genius. And it works to kill *billions* of cancer cells.

Dan C. Roehm, MD, a well-known oncologist and former cardiologist studied Dr. Budwig's protocol in 1990. Here are his comments:

> This diet is far and away the most successful anticancer diet in the world. What Dr. Johanna Budwig has demonstrated to my initial disbelief, but lately to my complete satisfaction in my practice, is this: Cancer is easily curable. The treatment is dietary, the response

is immediate; the cancer cell is weak and vulnerable; the precise biochemical breakdown point was identified by her in 1951, and is specifically correctable, in vitro as in vivo.[10]

Robert Wilner, MD, adds

A top European cancer research scientist, Dr. Johanna Budwig, has discovered a totally natural formula that protects against the development of cancer. Furthermore, people all over the world who have been diagnosed with incurable cancer and sent home to die have actually been cured and now lead normal, healthy lives.[11]

I mix the flaxseed oil with the cottage cheese and drink it every day. But beware: I have seen some overly complicated recipes for the mix. You have to do it right. Bill Henderson has simplified all this for those he coaches, and I follow his directions explicitly. I add water, but no sweetener. I'm happy with the taste and am committed to use it the rest of my life.

Let's make this simple. All you need to do is:

(1) Add 1/3 cup flax seed oil and 2/3 cup cottage cheese in a blender.

(2) Shake well.

(3) Wait 5 to 8 minutes.

(4) Add water, berries or nuts, if you wish.

(5) Blend at high speed for about 60 seconds.

(6) Drink immediately.

Of course, other ways to get more oxygen into our bodies exist. There is a problem, however, which I mentioned earlier. More oxygen in the blood does not necessarily mean more oxygen in the interior of our cells. And that's the key. Oxygen must permeate the cell membrane and get inside the cells.

Nevertheless, let's look at several inexpensive ways we get more oxygen into our bodies. Any increase improves overall health.

According to Warburg, a slightly alkaline pH in the body meant higher levels of oxygen uptake.

---

[10] Bill Henderson, Online Publishing & Marketing, LLC, Lexington, VA 2012.
[11] Online Publishing & Marketing, LLC, Lexington, VA 2012. Adapted from the Budwig Center in Spain and from Bill Henderson, one of my mentors.)

Certain fruits and berries such as blueberries and raspberries increase the body's uptake of oxygen. In fact, any food containing antioxidants is said to improve the oxygen levels in blood.

Essential fatty acids increase the amount of oxygen the hemoglobin in the bloodstream can carry. Essential fatty acids—omega-3s, omega-6s, and omega-9s cannot be produced in the human body, but we cannot live without them. (That's why they are called "essential.") These must be supplied in our diet. Flaxseed and meat, milk, and eggs from grassfed animals are rich sources of omega-3 fatty acids.

It should go without saying to avoid tobacco, alcohol, and drugs.

Fresh air helps. Stale air, carbon monoxide, numerous other gaseous fumes, and some chemicals interfere with the amount of oxygen the body takes in and sends to the bloodstream.

Exercise is a key to health, as we all know. While at Portland State College and Pacific Lutheran University, I competed in the mile, two-mile, and half-mile events. By daily practice, both sprints and long distance running, athletes are able to keep increasing lung capacity. (My best time for the mile was 4:18, which at that time was highly competitive, not long before world-class runners started breaking the 4-minute-mile barrier.) During training I experienced how rapidly lung capacity can increase through exercise.

Singing works too. Somewhere in my youthful training I can remember a choir instructor exhorting his choir members to "breathe deeply from the diaphragm in order to hold the long notes."

Meditation and relaxation reduce stress and help us "catch our breath" both literally and figuratively.

Proper (normal) breathing helps. Breathe from the diaphragm. Sometimes this is called "belly breathing." I know quite a bit about this because when I got pain from cancer and shingles my abdomen hurt just below the rib cage. To alleviate the pain I tended to bend over slightly. This, in turn, compacted my lungs and restricted normal breathing. When I straighten up, I get fuller breaths and feel healthier and stronger.

Good posture encourages normal breathing. The University of Missouri–Kansas City reports that improper breathing may reduce blood oxygen levels by 20 percent. Shallow breathing also reduces the amount of oxygen carried in the bloodstream. Improve your posture to increase energy, cleanse the lungs, and allow greater oxygen in the blood through proper breathing.

Doctors have often tested the oxygen levels in my blood. They use a simple device called a fingertip oximeter. When clipped onto a finger or toe it tells the oxygen level in the blood. For me the oximeter always reads about 99%, which is excellent. But how to get the hemoglobin to deliver the oxygen to the interior of the cells? That's the crucial question.

I, for one, along with cancer survivors worldwide, am thankful to Dr. Johanna Budwig. She found an answer.

I consider oxygenation of top-notch importance, yet it's not the only silver bullet worth firing from our arsenal. For months, I was in a quandary regarding the subject of alkalization. Why is it controversial? If it's valid, I didn't want to neglect it. If proper alkalization of the body is a hoax, get me away! Ultimately, a quote from Dr. Darrel Wolfe, the "Doc of Detox" got me off the fence. The next chapter reveals his exact words.

Chapter 6

Sixth Key: Be Wise—Alkalize!

While I was recovering from my first chemotherapy treatment, a man named Rodney and his wife came to our house. I was lying down, barely able to sit up when they arrived. Rod spoke passionately about the benefits of alkalizing my body as a treatment for cancer. Perhaps I'd heard the word "alkalization" in high school chemistry, but after all this time, I remembered little about what it meant.

Rodney explained that the United States had nuked the Japanese to end World War II and the Japanese had developed alkalizing as a means of neutralizing the effects of radiation in order to survive. I didn't understand much about what he was saying and was too sick to research the topic. Besides, I was already in chemo treatments and could not very well stop. Rod volunteered to bring me gallon jugs of alkalized water from his machine every day, which he did for some weeks.

Other people advised me that alkaline water as cancer therapy was one huge hoax. I was ignorant and had to put the matter on the shelf until later.

As it turns out, Rodney was "right on" about much of what he said.

What is "alkalization"? Let's imagine two extremes. One is a can of Coca Cola. The other is Drano, the household drain cleanser. Coke is extremely acidic and measures about 3.0 on the pH scale. Household cleaners such as Drano are extremely alkaline and measure about 14 on the pH scale. Spring water is about 7.0 on the scale and is termed neutral. Anyone knowledgeable about the effect of pH on the human body would be out of their mind to drink either Coke or Drano!

The pH scale measures how acidic or basic (alkaline) a substance is. It ranges from 0 to 14. A pH lower than 7 indicates the substance is an acid. If it is above 7 it is base or alkaline. Again, if pH is 7 it is neutral. pH stands for "potential hydrogen," and is defined as "the measurement of electrical resistance between negative and positive ions in the body."

Acidity and alkalinity are measured with a logarithmic scale. This means that something measuring 6 on the pH scale is 10 times more acidic than spring water. Something on the pH scale measuring 5 is 100 times more acidic than spring water, and so on.

Does that help? Probably not, unless you're a chemist. For the majority of us, let's look at it this way. Positive ions are acid forming and negative ions are alkalizing. There is a push and pull effect between the positive and negative ions. The pH measurement looks at how the ions push and pull against each other.

Knowing a bit more about the pH scale can help us arrive at better health. What is the optimum pH level for the human body? We should strive for a pH level of approximately 7.43, which is the normal pH level of our blood.

Every organ and tissue in the human body is affected by the pH level. Alternative doctors and researchers commonly understand and teach that healthy tissues and cells thrive in a neutral or slightly alkaline environment; that is, with a pH of 7 or slightly higher. These same doctors and researchers teach that diseases of all sorts—cancer, allergies, headaches, and weight problems—thrive in an acidic environment, that is, with a body pH of less than 7. Part of the reason the body thrives and diseases are driven away in an alkaline environment is because negative ions (-OH) are able to deliver more oxygen to the cells.

Fortunately, our bodies contain alkaline reserves and will fight to re-balance any deviations of fluctuating levels. However, the reserves are limited and in order to keep them intact it is important to eat the right kinds of foods—that is, alkalizing foods. The excess of alkali from alkalizing foods can be stored to neutralize acids in the future.[12]

Just how important is alkalization?

> *Every single person who has cancer has a pH that is too acidic.*
>
> —Dr. Darrell Wolfe, "Doc of Detox"

---

[12] http://www.healthextremist.com/top-7-alkalizing-foods-and-all-about-alkalizing-your-body (last accessed June 6, 2015).

That statement shook me to the core. It still shakes me every time I read it. If we can help people alkalize their bodies, we can help them avoid or heal from cancer and many other diseases. Although some medical personnel disregard this, those who are actually curing cancer generally agree: disease does not thrive in an alkaline environment.

How Can We Get Our Bodies Alkaline and Keep Them That Way?

Drink a lot of water every day. How much? No one really knows. Everybody is different, but it's commonly asserted 8 eight-ounce glasses per day is about right. Water helps flush acidic waste from the body.

The same is true with physical exertion. Brisk daily exercise helps flush out acidic waste from the body.

Breathe deeply. The added oxygen helps cleanse the body of acidic waste.

Take smaller bites at the table and chew food well. Saliva is alkaline. By eating slowly and chewing food well, a person can produce two gallons of highly alkaline liquid per day. Formerly, I could scarf down an entire meal in ten minutes. Since getting cancer and intentionally alkalizing my body, I try to take time to eat slowly and chew longer. I often take about an hour to eat a simple meal. I'm invariably the last one to finish eating.

How long does it take to thoroughly chew a medium bite of carrot? About a minute and a half. How long for a round slice of cucumber? Over a minute. And a slice of Roma tomato? About forty-five seconds. And don't even ask about celery! (The answer is forever and ever. Amen.)

You might think this matter about chewing food more fully is ridiculous. And it is if you start timing it. But hey! I had cancer and I don't want to get it again. My life depends on these little things. Dr. Darrell Wolfe preaches this mantra: Drink your solids and chew your liquids.

- Eliminate sugar, sugar substitutes, and junk food. I understand it takes a minimum of 30 glasses of water to neutralize the acidity of just one can of soda.

- Eliminate tobacco and alcohol since both are acidic.

- Emotional or psychological stress causes acidosis. Obviously, we need to relax, meditate, and eliminate stress where possible.

- Toxic overload from soil, water, and air pollution cause acid buildup in the body. Avoid pollution where possible.

- Barley or wheat grass supplements positively affect body pH levels.

- Mix a teaspoon of baking soda in a glass of water before or during each meal. Baking soda is dirt-cheap. You can't find a less expensive method of alkalizing than baking soda.

Diet affects the pH level of the body. In general, eat acidic foods and get an acidic body, although there are exceptions. Eat an alkaline diet, and get a healthy alkaline body.

Many helpful and colorful charts are available on the internet and in books which tell the pH level of specific foods. By way of illustration and reminder, avocadoes, apple cider vinegar, Swiss chard, tomatoes, lemon, raisins, and kale are alkaline in the body. (Note: everyone knows lemons are highly acidic. But lo and behold! When metabolized by the body, they have an alkaline effect.)

On the other hand, soft drinks, cheese, white bread, meat, canned tuna, and low-fat yogurt all promote acidity in the body. Charts differ. For example, Dr. David Williams lists milk, cream, and eggs as alkaline forming. Others suggest these same foods are acid forming. What gives? Why the disagreements? Various ways of testing reveal different pH levels. The science of testing pH levels of food is still developing.

Believe it or not, I practice all the above methods of alkalizing on a daily basis. It's rare for me to miss any. It's taken time. I muff it sometimes when I get in a rush and I'm still working at it, yet each of these practices are becoming second nature for me. A word for the healthy man: Be wise—alkalize!

While some controversy remains over the significance of alkalizing for optimum health, there is universal acceptance of the importance of the fascinating topic of the next chapter, our immune system. Without it, we would all be sick!

Chapter 7

Seventh Key: Marshall the World's Greatest Army—Your Immune System

Your immune system is one of the most marvelous and complex systems of the human body. It is composed of the skin, mucosal linings of body openings such as the nose, and internal organs such as the liver, kidneys, and spleen. Bone marrow and lymph glands are major players. The largest organ of all in the immune system is the digestive tract, which comprises 80% of the entire system.

Many knowledgeable people are aware of how the immune system is akin to an army and have described it in military terms. Here I quote Timothy Smith, MD in his intriguing article, "Your Incredible Immune Army":

> Your immune army uses an amazing array of weapons to protect you from cancer and microbes.
>
> There are good guys (our white blood cells) and bad guys (cancer and microorganisms) in us, and they are fighting it out for control of the territory that is you. I am going to put you in front of a powerful microscope so you can see—in vivid detail—this constant vicious struggle going on inside every one of us: the opposing armies, all manner of weapons including, guns, bombs, death ray guns, bioweapons, booby traps, missile defense systems, deceptive military maneuvers, and a communication system to die for—an unbelievably fantastic and unimaginably small but very real array of war machinery.
>
> The bad guys—the foreign invaders—are constantly attacking us; I speak of allergens, infectious agents, various toxins, and cancer. Our immune army, our guardian, is comprised of dozens of cell types with hundreds of different functions. In any single person,

immune cells number in the hundreds of billions—several times more than the number of stars in our galaxy or galaxies in our universe! They routinely sacrifice their teeny (but incredibly complex) lives to defend us.

Healthy immune cells are essential to our survival in this ongoing war, and they are relentless in their pursuit of cancer and other foreign invaders. When activated, they make Hitler, Stalin, and Mao look like neighborhood bullies. Immune cells attack in extremely large numbers—far larger than any army ever. Come to think of it, every single human has far more immune warriors than all the armies in history put together. Their onslaught is superbly coordinated by an extremely sophisticated communication and command system; human military intelligence operations are kindergarten games in comparison. Using a complex language comprised of molecular words (proteins, glycoproteins, cytokines, cell-signaling molecules, neurotransmitters, etc.), your immune cell soldiers release a barrage of chemical messages that identify foreign invaders, provide their location, estimate numbers, and coordinate the attack.

And what an awesome attack! Our immune cells sport an arsenal that would make Star Wars look puny. Immune cells can blow up enemy invaders. They can shoot out beams of ionized particles that literally rip holes in the outer cell membranes of infectious microbes and cancer cells. They release spurts of corrosive chemical poisons. They surround, cannibalize, and digest enemy cells—and then recycle the parts. They launch guided missiles from great distances that land and explode with incredible precision. They even smother their enemies in sticky goo (called complement) like the Marshmallow Man in Ghostbusters.

Your immune army deploys these remarkable weapons in multiple wars on several fronts. The skin, respiratory system, intestinal tract and bloodstream sustain the largest exposures and thus contain the most immune cells. Our largest exposure to pathogens—by far— is in the gut. Because this is the largest and most frequently breached barrier, roughly 80% of your white blood cells are embedded just beneath the intestinal mucosal surface. Microbes— in the form of bacteria, fungi, parasites, viruses, and the occasional helminth — are persistently knocking on the door and must be fended off on a non-stop basis. As you will see, we fend with some pretty big sticks. Imagine an army with hundreds of billions of white blood cell soldiers, each fully-equipped to take on cancer cells, viruses, and bacteria *mano a mano* in a struggle to the death.

Cancer cells are forming continuously in all of us, but alert, activated… immune cells will give them the instantaneous hatchet. If you're constantly vigilant and aggressively protective immune system took a coffee break, you'd be dead by the time it was over.[13]

What an exciting description! Want to learn more?

What Are Immune System Builders?

I passed by an Army Recruiting Station recently. The signs out front advertised how a common recruit could be turned into a formidable fighting machine. Military training videos invited, "Just sign up and you will become a man or woman of focus and force, a defender of freedom in a dangerous world. Training will transform you as part of an indestructible force."

The fact is, a strong military can be developed. The same is true of our personal defense unit to fight disease, pathogens, parasites, and whatever else attacks us to destroy us.

What are some Immune system builders? There are some surprises here. Who would think that sunshine could develop the military? Yet the vitamin D in sunshine is a powerful immune system builder. Get sunshine, not sunburn. Others include:

- Get plenty of sleep
- Manage your stress levels
- Meditate
- Talk in tongues (see Acts 2:1-21 in the Holy Bible). Research by Dr. Peterson at Oral Roberts Hospital indicates that use of the spiritual gift of tongues increased the immune system as much as exercise.
- Ingest sufficient amounts of real salt

---

[13] http://gcmaf.timsmithmd.com/book/chapter/12 (last accessed May 5, 2015).

- Stimulate the immune system. This can be done artificially by vaccinations or naturally by getting a cold or disease and fighting it off.

Then there are some not-so-surprising immune system builders:

- Eat your veggies, fruits, nuts, and seeds
- Get your exercise
- Take immune-building supplements
- Drink green tea extract
- Ingest adequate levels of minerals

What are immune system busters? If possible, avoid the following:

- Nicotine—both first- and second-hand tobacco smoke
- Excessive alcohol consumption
- Negative stress and emotions
- Toxins from heavy metals, such as copper and lead
- Sugars and artificial sweeteners
- Chemotherapy and radiation treatments
- Antibiotics and many medications
- Improper hormonal balance, such as a low level of iodine

What's So Great About the Immune System?

Amazingly, the immune system has a memory! If it battles a disease once, the entire system is prepared and ready to fight that specific disease again. For example, if a child catches measles, the system remembers and does not allow a second occurrence later in life.

To demonstrate the significance of the immune system, let me cap this chapter with quotes from Ty Bollinger's 11-part video series, *The Truth About Cancer: A Global Quest*.

> You can't have cancer if you have an intact immune system. If you have cancer, you can't have an intact immune system.—Rashid Buttar, MD

> Cancer is a result of a compromised immune system.—Unknown

Cancer is a disease of the immune system.—Keith Scott Mumby, MD

If you have a fully functioning immune system, you cannot have cancer.—Ty Bollinger, cancer researcher

The one thing that does cure cancer is your immune system.—Roby Mitchell, MD

Antibiotics don't heal; they can reduce the load of fungi, parasites, bacteria, etc., so the immune system can take over to heal.—Unknown

Doctors don't heal. The immune system heals.—Bob Wright, MD

The American Cancer Society states, "95% of all cancers are caused by environmental toxins." God designed our immune system to fight these toxins.

So much has been written about diet that I wondered if I could add anything to the subject. But when I suffered and nearly died from cancer, I knew I had some important messages about diet, nutrition, and the way foods are prepared. I realized the unsuspecting world needed to hear what I was learning.

Chapter 8

Eighth Key: Diet, Nutrition, and Cooking— Who's in Charge, Mouth or Mind?

More than any previous time in history, people recognize that diet and nutrition play significant roles in health. Still, many of us are discombobulated about what to eat and what not to eat. I chose that word purposefully. Most people are perplexed (confused, bewildered) about what "discombobulated" means. And that's the way it is with our attitude about what we place in our mouths.

Consider this dialogue.

Mouth: "I'd love to taste this cupcake."
Mind: "Oh, but you know you shouldn't."
Mouth: "Well, it's a small one with only a bit of frosting."
Mind: "You've already had enough for lunch."
Mouth: "I know, but Aunt Tillie gave us these cupcakes. I don't want to offend her."
Mind: "I don't either, but we are trying to shed a pound."
Mouth: "I'll just go ahead. Just this once. And besides, I'll eat less tonight."
Mind: (No comment)
Mouth: "Um, mmmm!"

So who's in charge here?

Eating is one of the pleasures of life. That's not bad, it's a good thing. Or shall we say, "It's a God thing." The Bible warns against *"men who forbid marriage and advocate abstaining from foods which God has created to be gratefully shared in by those who believe and know the truth. For everything created by God is good, and nothing is to be rejected if it is received with gratitude; for it is sanctified by means of the word of God and prayer"* (1 Timothy 3:3-5).

So food is good and God wants us to enjoy what we put into our mouths. But whatever we swallow has consequences.

There's no lack of advice and information about foods. Thank God for the digital age! If all the information—the good, the bad, and the ugly—were written on paper, I suppose every tree on earth would be required to produce the paper to print it.

The Healthiest People on Earth?

What foods promote health and healing? Take a peek at the natives of Kitava, one of the Trobriand Islands in Papua New Guinea. There folks are sometimes called "the healthiest people in the world." Why? Because disease was virtually non-existent among the denizens of the island.

The islanders have been subjects of extensive research. The well-known Malinowski study of the last century found that of the 23,000 people living on the island, there was not one single instance of heart disease, obesity, high blood pressure, dementia, stroke, or diabetes. Imagine that. Not a single instance of these killer diseases!

So how were the Kitavans living and eating differently than the rest of us? What was their secret to such incredible health? Over 30% of their diet consisted of fat! Yet none of the inhabitants were overweight, none suffered from acne, none had high blood pressure.

Dr. Malinowski died way back in 1942. Does his research into the Kitavian diet remain germane for us today?

Here's a quote from a current writer and researcher, Keith Scott-Mumby, MD, in his book *Diet Wise:* "[Conventional] doctors have it drummed into them that fats are bad for us. Whereas in fact certain fats are essential to survival and form part of our all-important cell membranes. Gosh, even our brains are forty percent fat; how would we even think without good clean fats?"

Dr. Michael A Schmidt authored *Smart Fats: How Dietary Fats and Oils Affect Mental, Physical and Emotional Intelligence.* He reports children in the womb and young children especially need abundant fats for normal brain development. After noting that our current dietary habits are "nearly devoid of fats critical to the brain," he makes further observations:

The normal brain cannot be made without omega-3 fatty acids. Purdue researchers found that individuals with symptoms of hyperactivity and attention deficit had lower levels of the omega-3 fatty acid DHA in their blood. Behavior and school performance as well as violence and aggression may also show a similar link to dietary fatty acids.

Learning problems, memory problems, mood disorders, behavior problems, tremors, numbness, developmental delays, seizures, stroke, autism, and other brain-related disorders have been corrected or improved by feeding appropriate fats and oils.

The Grassfed Revolution

Another factor we must consider concerning nutrition and diet is the difference between different kinds of meat. I'm not referring to the difference between meat from beef or pork or lamb. I'm referring to the major differences between meat from grassfed animals and grain-fed animals.

You think meat is meat, right? Not so fast. Think about it this way. We all know the difference between a slice of Sunbeam bread made from enriched white flour compared to a slice of whole grain bread like grandma used to bake. Press the white bread between your fingers and what do you get? A paper-thin sheet that is barely recognizable as bread. Now squeeze the whole grain bread between your thumb and forefinger and you still have recognizable bread. Anybody can see and feel the difference, yet we call them both "bread."

Now consider a steak from a grassfed steer and a steak from a grain-fed steer. The differences are mostly in nutrition, although a trained eye may spot the difference. The two look nearly identical. The grain-fed meat generally has more marbling (fat) throughout.

Grassfed beef is better for human health than grain-fed beef in ten different ways, according to the most comprehensive analysis to date. The 2009 study was a joint effort between the USDA and researchers at Clemson University in South Carolina. Compared with grain-fed beef, grassfed beef was:

- Lower in total fat
- Higher in beta-carotene
- Higher in vitamin E (alpha-tocopherol)
- Higher in the B-vitamins thiamin and riboflavin

- Higher in the minerals calcium, magnesium, and potassium
- Higher in total omega-3s, which fight cancer and heart disease
- A healthier ratio of omega-6 to omega-3 fatty acids (1.65 vs 4.84)
- Higher in CLA (cis-9 trans-11), a potential cancer fighter
- Higher in vaccenic acid (which can be transformed into CLA)
- Lower in the saturated fats linked with heart disease[14]

As for the health benefits of milk from grassfed cows, here's a report from Jo Robinson, New York Times best-selling author:

> For decades, we've been told that eating full-fat dairy products increases the risk of heart attack. Now, a study from the Journal of Clinical Nutrition says that the more full-fat dairy products people consume, the lower their risk of heart attack—provided the cows were grass-fed.
>
> The reason grassfed milk is protective is that it has up to five times more conjugated linoleic acid or CLA. CLA is a healthy fat found in the meat and milk of grazing animals. People who eat grass-fed dairy products absorb the CLA and store it in their tissues. In this study of over 3,500 people, those with the highest levels of CLA in their tissues had a fifty percent lower risk of heart attack than those with the lowest levels. Keeping Bossy on grass could prevent more heart attacks than putting people on expensive pharmaceutical drugs with all their troubling side effects. [15]

(Full Disclosure: Our family has been raising and marketing grassfed lamb since 1995.)

Why is all this significant? For a couple of reasons. First, any number of past studies have linked eating meat, especially red meat, with health problems such as heart disease, high cholesterol, obesity, and so forth. *Yet all*

---

[14] S. K. Duckett et al, *Journal of Animal Science*, June 2009, "Effects of winter stocker growth rate and finishing system on: III. Tissue proximate, fatty acid, vitamin, and cholesterol content." http://www.eatwild.com/news.html (last accessed April 27, 2015).

[15] L. A. Smit, A. Baylin, and H. Campos, 2010, "Conjugated linoleic acid in adipose tissue and risk of myocardial infarction." *The American Journal of Clinical Nutrition*. http://www.eatwild.com/news.html (last accessed April 27, 2015).

of these studies are based on the meat from grain-fed animals. Not one that I'm aware of at this writing is based on meat from grassfed animals!

Second, meat from grassfed animals is actually loaded with omega-3 fatty acids and is healthful for humans. Lab studies indicate the CLA from grassfed meat can actually eliminate cancer cells! Avoiding meat—that is, meat from grazing animals—may be hazardous for your health!

Third, the Bible promotes and in some cases, commands the eating of meat. Think of the Passover meal, which consists of lamb. As for milk, how could a good God bring His chosen people into a land "flowing with milk and honey," only for people to later determine that milk is harmful to the body?

We need to respect each person's choices. Each human body is complex beyond comprehension. What's best for one man or one woman may not be the right choice for others. Let each one be convicted in his own mind.

Cooking

The importance of cooking and food preparation cannot be overlooked. For many years I owned and managed the number-one rated (on Google) niche website for www.grassfedrecipes.com. The site is filled with recipes and healthful cooking tips. Here are some of my favorites.

1. Cook low and slow.

When it comes to roast recipes, I admit I was startled. Shocked. Flabbergasted might be most accurate.

I read in Adelle Davis's *Let's Cook It Right*, "In experiments where identical roasts were cooked at different oven temperatures to the same degree of doneness, roasts cooked for 26 to 32 hours were preferred in 100 per cent of the taste tests to roasts cooked in 3 hours or less."

Although I was skeptical, we went ahead and tried it. Adelle proved to be absolutely right!

The meat was amazingly delicious. It was juicy, tender, and not dried out at all. Savory meat easily peeled off the bone. This slow-cooked recipe for roast lamb has to be a supreme choice for any roast. It will work for pot roast lamb, lamb shoulder roast, or any other lamb roast.

> ### All-Day, All-Night Lamb Roast Recipe
>
> Procedure: Set the oven temperature to 170 degrees F. Set the roast in a pan, cover, and place in the oven.
>
> It requires no watching; it can't burn. In addition, vitamins and minerals can't be harmed at such a low temperature. Almost no fuel is required to cook it. The fat in the lamb meat will slowly cook out so you end up with a fat-free roast lamb recipe.
>
> The exact cooking time is not significant. Allow plenty of time. (See above.) We were startled at how tender and savory this recipe for roast lamb became. I think you will be too.

2. Cooking and processing destroys vitamins and minerals.

With his characteristic humor with a message, Dr. Darrel Wolfe says, "The more you cook, the worse you look." And "The more you fry, the sooner you die."

I understand most vitamins and minerals are found just under the skins. Even peeling potatoes or carrots removes the most nutrient-rich area.

3. Eat food in the most natural, unprocessed state possible.

Eat Raw? One day a man called and wanted to buy a grassfed lamb bundle. He explained he ate raw because he was trying to overcome cancer. Eating raw had not yet become the craze it is today. I was appalled by the idea of eating raw meat, or anything else raw for that matter.

Later, I thought about it. We all eat uncooked carrots, lettuce, celery, tomatoes and a nearly unlimited number of other veggies. We eat bananas, apples, grapes, and most other fruits in a natural state. It also dawned on me that nearly every morning at that time I drank an eggnog with raw eggs and didn't think it strange.

So how about raw meat and other foods? I generally order steaks not well done nor even medium. I prefer steaks "rare" with a ribbon of pink inside.

The point is, rare or raw is not so bad and may even be healthier than we think. Consider this quote from Joel Wallach, MD, author of the famous *Dead Doctors Don't Lie* treatise (over 170 million copies are in print). "Ladies, according to University double-blind placebo controlled studies, you reduce your breast cancer potential by 462% just by cooking your meat medium rare instead of well done."[16]

4. Avoid vegetable oils. Instead, cook with coconut oil or natural fat.

5. Be aware that microwave cooking destroys vitamins and minerals.

6. Beware of salad dressings.

I have observed that people who claim to love salads really love the dressings more than the salads. How many folks do you know who eat salads without dressing? It makes no sense to try to lose weight by choosing a salad and then loading it up with umpteen calories in a dressing.

For me, the best salad dressing is … surprise—applesauce! Tastes great on most any salad!

By the way, please let me know what is helpful to you in this book. I'm looking for more "cancer survivor" stories. I'm available at BMarkAnderson.com. And by all means, get this information into the hands of people you know who have been diagnosed with cancer! Better yet, give them this book *before* they get cancer or any other disease. You could well save the life of someone you care about. I only wish the truth had come to me before I got sick.

7. Eat slowly, take smaller bites, and chew food longer.

Your mother probably used to say "Chew your food longer." Now we know why. Chewing produces saliva and saliva produces enzymes necessary for digestion. Digestion gets the nutrients where we need them. Undigested food becomes fecal waste in the intestines.

Fecal waste? Most of us prefer to avoid the subject. Yet, it's a key to overcoming many cancers and it's the eye-opening topic of the next chapter.

---

[16] http:www.americanaci.org (last accessed May 25, 2015).

Chapter 9

Ninth Key: Detox or Die—Slogan for the 21st Century

Detoxification is more important than I ever imagined. I used to see detox ads and scorned them as a hoax. No more. As several oncologists reveal in Ty Bollinger's video series *The Truth About Cancer: A Global Quest*, detox is essential to overcoming cancer.

What is detoxification? Detox is simply the removal of poisons or toxins from the body or mind. Why is detox becoming so important? Consider these statements:

> 95% of all cancers are caused by environmental toxins.—American Cancer Society

> Over 80% of all illnesses have environmental and lifestyle causes.—United States Center for Disease Control[17]

> There was a study where they took 10 newborn infants and measured the umbilical cord blood for toxins. There were 287 toxic chemicals found on average: 208 were carcinogenic.—David C. Jockers, DC

> For some, dental cavitation and root canals are a surprising and overlooked cause of cancer: Dentistry plays an enormous role, 95% of females with breast cancer have a dental involvement.—Burton Goldberg, Author, Lecturer

---

[17] http://medicaldictionary.thefreedictionary.com/Detoxification (last accessed May 7, 2015).

A study completed in 1923 by over 60 dentists concluded there is no safe way to perform a root canal.—Bill Henderson, Lecturer, Author, Cancer Coach[18]

What are these environmental toxins that affect nearly everyone on the planet? Herbicides, insecticides, fluorides, chlorines, household cleaners, heavy metals such as copper, arsenic, chemicals or metals in women's makeup, antibiotics, some medicines, agricultural or industrial chemicals, and synthetic hormones. Then there are the pollutants from PCBs, electrical pollution from computer screens, tablets, and cell phones. GMOs are guilty according to many experts.

Parasites, bacteria, viruses, infections, yeast (think candida) and diseases (such as Lyme disease), chemicals from medical treatments including surgery, chemotherapy, radiation, X-rays, MRIs, and PET scans all contribute. The list never seems to end.

While the technician prepped me for a CAT scan, I asked her, "What are the long-term effects of this CAT scan you are giving me?" "They cause cancer twenty years from now," she replied succinctly, and walked away. I noticed she stepped out of the room for the duration of every test.

Stress, especially unhealthful anxiety, produces toxins.

In addition, our bodies produce toxins. The most compelling article I've read on the subject of detoxification is "Spoiled Rotten" by Dr. Darrell Wolfe, the "Doc of Detox." He states that the average person carries about twelve pounds of undigested fecal matter in his or her intestines, mainly in the colon. This renders the colon "comatose" and allows toxins to leak out into the blood stream and into surrounding tissues and organs. It's a source of "leaky gut syndrome" which causes myriad types of sickness and disease.

A comatose or malfunctioning colon affects the liver. The liver can't keep up with its job of removing toxins from the blood. When the liver becomes overwhelmed, the burden passes on to the kidneys, which are not designed to do what the liver is supposed to do. The domino effect continues throughout the digestive system, negatively affecting our entire well-being.

According to Dr. Wolfe, most diseases start in the colon. Why is it that prostate cancer in men and ovarian cancer in women are so common? Because these organs reside in close proximity to the colon. Restore the colon

---

[18] http://www.cancertutor.com/quest-for-cures-dirty-dozen-prevent-cancer (last accessed May 19, 2015).

and many diseases never have a chance to gain a foothold. Detoxification to restore this organ is essential for health.

Let's Talk About Parasites

The Center for Disease Control (CDC) warns that millions in the US are infected with parasites. More than 60 million persons are chronically infected with *Toxoplasma gondii*. Each year 1.1 million people are newly infected with *Trichomonas*.[19]

Parasites are controversial. We think only people in Third World countries are infected. Think again. One medical doctor who specializes in parasitology notes 96% of all Americans carry parasites.

A parasite is an organism that lives on or in a host organism and gets its food from or at the expense of its host. They need us but we don't need them.

Keith Scott Mumby, MD, MB ChB, PhD, rates as one of the world's top experts in parasitology. He has a lot of critical information regarding parasites:

> In "The Body Snatchers," *National Geographic* reported, "Parasites have killed more humans than all the wars in history" [Season 1, episode 17].
>
> Parasites are all around us: in the air we breathe, the food we eat and the water we drink. Every single living organism can be infected by these super-beasts.
>
> 4.5 billion worms exist. They can be found in both unsanitary and sanitary conditions, around the globe. So if you were thinking that you didn't have to worry because you live in America, Japan, Germany etc, and in sanitary conditions, you would be wrong. Very wrong.
>
> For example, around 40 million people in the United States are infected with the *Enterobiasis* pinworm. Pinworms affect an estimated 5.5 million children within the United States.
>
> Most people think that if you are clean living and take precautions, like frequent hand washing, you won't get parasites. That's not

---

[19] http://www.cdc.gov/parasites/npi/index.html (last accessed May 19, 2015).

true. You can pick up an egg or cyst anywhere. Just touch a doorknob and you could pick up an egg. Just one egg can kill you!

There is a well-known medical history of a strict, clean-living, orthodox Jew from New York. He was admitted to hospital with what's called a "space occupying lesion" in the skull. That usually means a tumor, starting to squeeze the brain and producing strange symptoms.

But when operated on, the neurosurgeon found a large growing cyst from a pork tapeworm. It was an easy, if revolting, cure and the man had cause to be thankful the diagnosis was as lenient as it was. But the striking part of this story is that the man never ate pork in his life … I mean ever!

He had touched a door knob or telephone or some other object at some time, which was infected with eggs. Probably touched his mouth or lips later and that was it: the worm was inside him and traveled to his skull. It only takes one egg to make a cyst the size of a baseball. This condition is called "cysticercosis".

The Myth: Parasites infect only dirty people and foreigners. This is the #1 myth and it is nonsense. You can pick up an infection on the slightest contact, such as water used to rinse your salad.

Get real. Parasites are rampant in the Western world, not just Third World countries.

Meat isn't so much a worry. Pork meat frozen at minus 30 degrees for a week or more will be cleared of all living *Trichinella*. The real danger is "fresh" produce, such as leaves, fruits and roots, which cannot be deep frozen.[20]

Diet Without Detoxification is Deception

About one-third of people globally are infected by just one type of parasite, *Toxoplasma gondii*. In parts of Europe, infection rates are as high as 90 percent, but in the United States, the average rate of infection falls between 10 percent and 20 percent. *Toxoplasma gondii*, which can live in our brains, has links to such psychiatric conditions as suicide attempts and schizophrenia.[21]

---

[20] http://parasites911.com/1sc (last accessed in May 2015).
[21] http://www.dana.org/Publications/Brainwork/Details.aspx?id=43808 (last accessed May 19, 2015).

As you can see, parasites are everywhere. No one is safe. These critters, some microscopic, some inches or feet long, can overwhelm the immune system of even a healthy individual and cause sickness, blindness, mental disorder, and death.

That's the bad news. The good news is detoxification can rid the body of parasites!

Diet gets a huge and well-deserved amount of attention these days. But when it comes to disease prevention, diet is only part of the picture. Diet without detoxification is deception. Both are essential as long as we live on a polluted planet.

Someone said it like this. "We are exposed to more toxins in a single day than our grandparents were in their entire lifetime."

Many forms of detoxification are possible. Some are complex and expensive; others are simple and cost pennies per day. I use Essiac tea which is not only a detoxification drink, but has killed cancer by itself for thousands of people. Essiac tea is a mixture of roots and herbs simmered together and can be purchased in health stores or over the internet. The four main ingredients are Burdock Root, Slippery Elm Inner Bark, Sheep Sorrel and Indian Rhubarb Root. I drink 1/3 cup daily.

Again, Detox or Die: Slogan for the 21st century.

To research cancer and how to conquer it can become overwhelming. There's so much complicated information out there. That's why I've tried to reduce matters to 9 essential keys. In an effort to make things plain and simple, let me summarize what I do. These are keys to maintain health and keep cancer at bay.

Chapter 10

Summary: Here's What I Do

Here's what I do—and what I suggest—to keep cancer away. I'm not saying my way is the only way, but it's working for me and thousands of others who try something similar. It's so simple you can write it on a 3x5 card. Do it to keep cancer away forever! I get no profit from any of the sources or links.

1. **Get a coach**. Webster Kerr, former webmaster at www.CancerTutor.com, was my original guide. He has tons of information and is especially astute at evaluating various protocols. We also chose Bill Henderson because he made things simple. His website is www.beating-cancer-gently.com.

2. **Meditate.** I intentionally take time to read, mull over, and (if no one is around) to softly voice God's healing truths from the Bible.

3. **Support group**. For me, it's my family and church. I couldn't keep eating a cancer-free diet without the support of my wife and family.

4. **Modern medicine**. I continue checkups with my oncologist, Dr. James Feeley.

5. **Budwig Diet**. Here's a simple recipe: Mix one-third cup flaxseed oil with two-thirds cup of cottage cheese. Shake up the mixture. Let it sit for five to eight minutes, then add a little water to suit your taste. Blend at a high speed in a blender. Drink immediately. I do this once every day. We buy flaxseed oil at our local HyVee grocery store, or you can buy it on the internet.

6. **Be wise—alkalize!** I discipline myself to eat vegetables (especially leafy greens) every meal. I swallow six or seven barley tablets about fifteen minutes before each meal. GreenSupreme not only has a great price, but gives pH strips for free to test pH levels when you order. Call 1-800-358-0777. I also take a teaspoon of baking soda stirred into a cup of water before or during each meal.

7. **Immune system.** I order Transfer Point Beta-1, 3D Glucan tablets from www.ancient5.com or 1-800-877-8220. My mentor advises one 500 mg tablet per 50 pounds weight every morning before breakfast. It's expensive. I also take about ½ teaspoon per day of XPC, a fermented yeast culture from cereal grains, as suggested by Dr. David Williams. Buy at pennies per day on eBay or www.4spectrum.us. Avoid alcohol, sugars, nicotine, and soda pop.

8. **Nutrition.** Supplements are essential to overcome cancer. I take mega doses of Vitamin D3. For two months I took 25,000 I.U. per day then reduced to 10,000 I.U. per day. www.PuritansPride.com supplies the gel capsules. I take a vitamin/mineral supplement twice a day called Daily Advantage from www.DrDavidWilliams.com. I take two capsules of Heart Plus and one capsule of Green Tea Extract with every meal. www.MakingHealthAffordable.com has an amazingly low price for those two products which work synergistically together. In addition, I am careful to avoid all forms of sugar. I avoid gluten and processed foods as much as possible.

9. **Detoxify daily**. Some prefer coffee enemas. I simply drink one-third cup of Essiac tea each day. Many sources for Essiac tea are available on the internet, including www.Starwest-Botanicals.com.

It seems like every week we hear of someone getting cancer. The American Cancer Society projects one out of every two men and one out of every three women alive today will get cancer in their lifetime. I have found an *Answer for Cancer*. If you want a speaker to come to your organization to give some hope, a little humor, and the inside story about cancer, let me know by contacting me at BMarkAnderson.com.

Give me a blender, flax oil, and some cottage cheese. I'll mix the Budwig Protocol before the eyes of your audience and tell why it's a cancer killer. You'll never have a presentation like it!

In Part One of this book I share my experience of healing. Part Two outlines nine natural and spiritual keys to prevent and cure cancer. One of these essentials involves meditation and confession of God's word. What is the role of God and His word in healing today? Part Three deals with the most important and often-overlooked action: the spiritual. It is the area of my expertise and the primary reason I am alive today.

Part Three

Meditation on God and His Word

> *For cancer patients my big recommendation is faith in God. Be strong with your spiritual part of your life.*
>
> —Dr. Tony Jimenez, MD

I was sick with cancer at the time, desperately needing help and hope. Then, as I explained in Chapter One, Greta Eubanks, my wife's cousin, sent us a photocopy of a folder containing four parallels between natural and spiritual medicine. As I read the little booklet, the idea of the parallels between natural medicine and the spiritual medicine of God's word began to send tidal waves through my entire being. A tsunami of hope swelled up inside me.

I didn't know it at the time, but after a months-long search I found Joyce Meyer's ministry had published the parallels and related verses on the internet. The copy I received was a compendium of healing scriptures and Holy Spirit-inspired confessions to go with them. I am free from cancer today in large part because of that little folder. I give credit to God and to Joyce Meyer's ministry for publishing those Scriptures.

The little folder contained several moving thoughts—literally life-transforming lines. In particular, this statement sounded a trumpet in my soul: "Listen, instead of wondering whether you have enough faith to be healed, just take the medicine."

Here's another striking sentence from that booklet. "We might say that medicine is no respecter of persons. It will work for anyone who takes it. It is not a matter if God is willing or not willing to heal any individual, but whether the individual will receive healing by taking the medicine that produces it." Reading that sentence began to set me free.

Wow! I was blown away! I needed these truths.

I read and reread the parallels, the Scriptures, and the related confessions. (I was so weak and sick I couldn't do much else!) I ruminated on the verses and they became my own, sometimes word for word. I digested them. I lived by them. They became my food and drink. *Your words were found and I ate them, and Your words became for me a joy and the delight of my heart* (Jeremiah 15:16). The words of the Almighty penetrated my spirit and affected healing in my mind and body. What His word did for me, He will do for you and anyone else who digests His words.

As I continued to meditate on these parallels and the associated Bible verses, other connections came to mind. I added four more parallels.

Many Godly Christians struggle with healing. We all know and grieve for someone who agonizes with pain and disease. Part Three of *Answer for Cancer: 9 Keys* can produce healing from God. Through His energizing word, God gives you the results for which you are waiting. What has eluded you in the past can now be yours.

You will not only be blessed as you meditate on the following truths—you will find the avenue of healing and health.

Chapter 11

God's Word is His Medicine

There are several parallels between God's medicine and natural medicine. God's word is a cure and a medicine to our whole body. Isaac Leeser's translation of Exodus 15:26 reads *I the Lord am thy physician*. The medicine the Great Physician prescribes is His word.

Many make the mistake of substituting belief in healing for the actual taking of God's prescribed medicine—His word. They say, "I believe in healing" without actually taking the medicine. What good would it do to believe in food if you didn't eat any? You would starve. What good would it do to believe in water if you didn't drink any? You would die of thirst.

The First Parallel: God's Word is a Healing Agent.

Just as natural medicine is a healing agent or catalyst, so is God's word. To say it another way, the medicine itself contains the capacity to produce healing. Inherent within God's word is the capacity, the energy, the ability, and the nature to effect healing in your body.

> **Isaiah 55:11** For as the rain and the snow come down from heaven, And do not return there without watering the earth And making it bear and sprout, And furnishing seed to the sower and bread to the eater; So will My word be which goes forth from My mouth; It will not return to Me empty, Without accomplishing what I desire, And without succeeding in the matter for which I sent it.

Every word of God has a specific purpose. It will accomplish what it was sent to do. The word contains the power to produce what it says. Just as when God said, "Let there be light" and there was light, healing Scriptures contain the capacity to produce healing. Just as raindrops activate the natural processes of soil, so healing words activate the natural healing processes of the body.

> **Hebrews 4:12** For the word of God is living and active and sharper than any two-edged sword, and piercing as far as the division of soul and spirit, of both joints and marrow, and able to judge the thoughts and intentions of the heart.

God's Message is full of life and power—Weymouth

God's word to us is something alive, full of energy—Knox

God's word is alive with energy—Jordan

The Second Parallel: Medicine is No Respecter of Persons

It will work for anyone who takes it. It is not a matter if God is willing or not willing to heal any individual, but whether the individual will receive healing by taking the medicine that produces it.

The Third Parallel: Medicine Must Be Taken According to Directions to Be Effective

Some medicine labels read, "Take internally"; others say, "Take externally." To rub a medicine on our body externally when the directions say to take it internally will not work. To take it after meals when the directions say to take it before meals will reduce its effectiveness. To take it once in a while when the directions say three times a day will give limited results, if any. No matter how good the medicine is, it must be taken according to the directions or it won't work. So it is with God's medicine; it must be taken according to directions for it to work.

The directions for taking God's medicine are found in Proverbs 4:20-22: *My son, give attention to my words; Incline your ear to my sayings. Do not let them depart from your sight; Keep them in the midst of your heart. For they are life to those who find them and health to all their body.*

Attending to God's words, inclining our ears to them, and keeping them before our eyes causes the word to get into the core of our being. It is only as His words get into our spirit (our heart) and stay there that they produce healing in our body. Head knowledge won't do. They must penetrate our spirit through meditation—attending, hearing, looking, muttering, musing, pondering—to produce healing in our body. However, once they do penetrate, they will surely bring health to all our whole body. Let them penetrate deep within your heart.

We can see again that God's way of healing is spiritual. Power is ministered first to our spirit, then distributed to our body. God's medicine must be taken internally. Listen, instead of wondering whether you have enough faith to be healed, just take the medicine. This book contains healing Scriptures. Feed on them several times a day, repeating them over and over again to yourself. The medicine will work if we get it inside of us.

The Fourth Parallel: Medicine Takes Time to Work

People give natural medicine a lot of time, patience, and money to work. They take the prescription back for refills and more refills. They are diligent about it. They don't just swallow one dose and expect a miracle. Keep taking God's medicine. Give it time to work.

The Fifth Parallel: Medicine is Expensive

Natural medicine costs money; spiritual medicine costs time. Face it: it takes time to meditate and get God's word into our spirit. This is how God planned it. He wants to spend His time with us. He takes pleasure in His people. Be honest. Is it worth your time in meditation with the Lover of your soul in order to receive healing?

If you choose to receive God's healing, take your medicine. Say these Scriptures aloud to yourself. Think about what you're saying in your heart. Use these confessions, and the ones you develop on your own, as praises to the Father. His word is medicine to every part of our body.

The Sixth Parallel: Medicine is Immensely Profitable

Natural medicines profit manufacturers, pharmacies, insurance companies, and the doctors who prescribe them. Medicine has a ripple effect throughout the industry.

God's word is also immensely profitable. Profitable, that is, for the one who ingests it. It produces physical, emotional, and spiritual effects in the one who feeds on it. In addition, God's word creates ripple effects. As His word heals, strengthens, and mollifies the one who takes the medicine, it also encourages, strengthens, and comforts those around. In fact, the positive ripple effects of God's word on the man or woman who receives healing may influence multitudes for salvation around the world!

The Seventh Parallel: All Medicine Has Side Effects

A recent prescription bottle came with a two-page printout that began "WARNING: May cause headache, nausea, dry mouth, sleepiness …." All the side effects listed were negative.

Meditating on God's word also carries side effects beyond the stated purpose. Praise God! All the side effects are positive. Greater sense of Divine Presence, inner peace, better sleep, becoming more Christ-like, more power, more love, and more patience are some of the common side effects of spending time drinking in God's word.

Don't diminish the side effects of God's medicine. In fact, these "secondary effects" are some of the most powerful reasons to meditate on God's word. They automatically produce the hoped-for qualities many strive for yet never attain. Perhaps Bibles ought to carry this message inside the front cover: "WARNING: May cause growth of the fruit of the Spirit. May cause more grace, more power to overcome temptation, may create emotional healing …."

The Eighth Parallel: Everyone Must Swallow His Own Medicine

I can't swallow your pills for you and you can't drink my medication for me. A caretaker can encourage, advise, cajole, instruct, and even organize the pill tray for another, but he or she cannot imbibe someone else's medication for them. Personal responsibility is the bottom line for both natural medicine and God's word. If you want the benefit, you've got to take the medicine.

God is a practical God. He may be mysterious, yet He is also down-to-earth and plain-spoken. Let's be specific. What exactly are the words that heal?

Chapter 12

God Heals You by His Word

Let me tell you a story about one of the specific words from God that was instrumental in my healing. It came after the second cancer diagnosis.

A cancer diagnosis leaves confusion. Why? How? Really? Is this even possible? My head was swimming. This was especially true for me because my body had responded well to the first set of chemo treatments. I thought I was "cured" by the chemotherapy. But now cancer had returned! And it was worse than before. What did I do to deserve this?

I was sinking deeper and deeper into sickness by the day. It wasn't that I had no hope. I simply didn't know where to turn or what to do.

About this time I read a Scripture that hit me like a ton of bricks. It was a well-timed silver bullet that killed doubt dead. I suppose every cancer patient turns introspective trying to discover what he did wrong to deserve such a terrible judgment. This verse from Galatians liberated me: *Christ redeemed us from the curse of the Law, having become a curse for us—for it is written, 'Cursed is everyone who hangs on a tree'* (Galatians 3:13).

When I read that verse I knew whatever I may or may not have done, I was freed. The curse was broken. Cancer had to go from my body. If I had done something in my past or present to bring cancer on my body, I didn't have to think about it any longer. Christ had set me free from the curse and consequences of the law! He Himself had absorbed the curse.

I expected healing to ensue at any time. That didn't happen outwardly, but the liberating word from God built a confidence into my innermost being that all sickness would go.

Additional specific healing promises encouraged me:

✟ ✟ ✟

Proverbs 4:20-22 My son, give attention to my words; Incline your ear to my sayings. Do not let them depart from your sight; Keep them in the midst of your heart. For they are life to those who find them And health to all their body.

20-22 My son, attend to my words; consent and submit to my sayings. Let them not depart from your sight; keep them in the center of your heart. For they are life to those who find them, healing and health to all their flesh. (AMP)

20-22 My son, pay attention to my words. Open your ears to what I say. Do not lose sight of these things. Keep them deep within your heart because they are life to those who find them and they heal the whole body. (NOG)

20-22 Dear friend, listen well to my words; tune your ears to my voice; Keep my message in plain view at all times. Concentrate! Learn it by heart! Those who discover these words live, really live; body and soul, they're bursting with health. (MSG)

22 For they are life unto every one of those that find them, and to all his body a healing. (Leeser)

22 For, life, they are, to them who find them,—and, to every part of one's flesh, they bring healing. (Rotherham)

MEDITATION: God's word is not lifeless. It's bursting with creative power. When You said, "Let there be light!" there was light and the darkness disappeared. You have spoken Your healing word into my life. Your creative word is in me now. Like a sponge, I'm absorbing Your healing life and word into my spirit. Your word is downloading into my spirit and flowing into each cell of my body. Cancer doesn't have a chance. Pain must go. I will never be the same again! Your word is creating health in every cell of my body. Germs, viruses, toxins, and every other cause of disease and cancer are leaving my body now.

✟ ✟ ✟

Psalm 107:20 He sent His word and healed them, And delivered them from their destructions.

20 He sent his word, and healed them, and delivered them from their destructions. (KJV)

20 He sendeth his word and healeth them, and delivereth them from their graves. (Leeser)

20 [H]e sent his word and healed them, he delivered them from destruction. (Stern)

20 He spoke the word that healed you, that pulled you back from the brink of death. (MSG)

20 He sent out His word, and it healed, and from their corruptions, it freed! (Fenton)

1 Thessalonians 2:13 … the word of God which also performs its work in you who believe.

13 [T]he word of God, which effectually worketh also in you that believe. (KJV)

MEDITATION: Lord, You have sent each word for a purpose. Your healing words contain healing energy. I'm absorbing that energy into my spirit as I meditate and digest Your word. That life-giving energy is now flowing into my body and causing healing. It's affecting every cell, every tissue in my body right now. Your word is effectively working and fulfilling the purpose for which you sent it. You are accomplishing Your pleasure in me. Your power is flowing through my personal spirit and healing my body and mind right now. Your word is freeing me from corruption and establishing me in perfect health.

✝ ✝ ✝

"At the cross, at the cross, where I first saw the light…" so goes the old hymn. When it comes to healing, we must invariably turn to the cross of Christ. There is healing at the cross.

Chapter 13

God Heals You by the Cross

I have never been one to focus on the accounts of the cross as recorded in the four gospels. The cross accounts are not pleasant to read because they are so graphic and gruesome. Besides, the chapters are long. I have tended to avoid these sections of Matthew, Mark, Luke, and John whenever possible.

This attitude changed when I began to believe God to heal me from cancer. Obviously, I had failed to fully appreciate the cross and God's purpose for the crucifixion. My understanding of the cross was largely focused on forgiveness of sin and the power to overcome the devil. While I had some idea and experience of sacrificing my life as Jesus did, my thinking of the cross was clearly immature.

My great need for healing opened the door to embracing the sufferings of Jesus in a fresh way. The cross became more personal for me. I needed the cross.

The more time I spend meditating on Christ, His suffering, and the predetermined purposes of the cross, the more I gravitate toward God. The cross explains to me how much God loves His creation. I'm hungry for God; I'm hungry for the cross. Today I embrace the cross. The cross makes "bitter waters sweet," and I love it!

✞ ✞ ✞

Exodus 15:25 Then he cried out to the LORD, and the LORD showed him a tree; and he threw it into the waters, and the waters became sweet. There He made for them a statute and regulation, and there He tested them.

25 And he cried unto the LORD; and the LORD shewed him a tree, which when he had cast into the waters, the waters were made sweet: there he made for them a statute and an ordinance, and there he proved them. (KJV)

MEDITATION: Lord, thank you for the cross (the tree). Thank you for the cross that makes bitter waters sweet. Thank you for the cross that separates the Old Covenant from the New Covenant, and my old life from my new life. I have been crucified with Christ. The cross has separated me from cancer, sin, sickness, Satan and the side-effects of cancer. Thank you for removing all pain, paralysis, and numbness from my body. Thank you that you have already made this separation and I'm on the resurrection side of the cross, never to return to the other side. Thank you for making me free, whole, and healthy because of the cross.

✞ ✞ ✞

Revelation 13:8 the Lamb slain from the foundation of the world. (NASB margin)

8 the Lamb slain from the foundation of the world. (KJV, YLT)

MEDITATION: Lord, in Your mind the crucifixion and all that went with it was planned and determined from the foundation of the world. The great benefits of Calvary were not left to chance. Justification, glorification, and healing were settled in heaven from the outset. I lay hold of my healing; I take what You planned for me from the beginning. Thank you for accomplishing Your predetermined plan—my healing!

✞ ✞ ✞

Isaiah 53:3-5 He was despised and forsaken of men, a man of sorrows (or pains) and acquainted with grief (or sickness); and like one from whom men hide their face He was despised, and we did not esteem Him.

Surely our griefs (or sickness) He Himself bore, And our sorrows (or pains) He carried; yet we ourselves esteemed Him stricken, smitten of God, and afflicted.

But He was pierced through for our transgressions, He was crushed for our iniquities; the chastening for our well-being fell upon Him, and by His scourging we are healed.

3 A man of pains, and acquainted with sickness … (YLT)

3 a man of pains, and acquainted with disease …. (Leeser)

3 a man of suffering who knew what sickness was. (HCSB)

4 Surely our sicknesses he hath borne, and our pains -- he hath carried them. (YLT)

4 Yet He Himself bore our sicknesses, and He carried our pains. (HCSB)

5 ... with his stripes we are healed. (KJV, DBY, WEB, HNB, ASV)

5 ... And by his bruise there is healing to us. (YLT)

5 ... and with his wounds we are healed. (ESV)

Matthew 8:16-17 When evening came, they brought to Him many who were demon-possessed; and He cast out the spirits with a word, and healed all who were ill. This was to fulfill what was spoken through Isaiah the prophet: "HE HIMSELF TOOK OUR INFIRMITIES AND CARRIED AWAY (OR REMOVED) OUR DISEASES."

17 ... He Himself took (in order to carry away) our weaknesses and infirmities and bore away our diseases. (AMP)

17 He took away our illnesses and lifted our diseases from us. (New English Bible)

MEDITATION: Lord, You took my sickness and my grief to the cross. You became my Scapegoat. You took my diseases, including cancer, into the wilderness, never for them to return. Since You took them, I refuse to have them. I refuse to accept any cancer cells in my body. I reject all cancer and its side effects. I refuse to accept in my body what You took in Your body. You took my pains and carried them away. Nothing shall by any means hurt me. You were beaten, bruised, smitten, lashed, wounded, and striped for me. By Your wounds, stripes, lashes, and bruises, I was healed now and forever.

☦ ☦ ☦

Galatians 2:20 I have been crucified with Christ; and it is no longer I who live, but Christ lives in me; and the life which I now live in the flesh I live by faith in the Son of God, who loved me and gave Himself up for me.

20 With Christ I have been crucified, and live no more do I, and Christ doth live in me; (YLT)

20 I have been crucified with Christ [in Him I have shared His crucifixion]; (AMP)

20 When the Messiah was executed on the stake as a criminal, I was too; so that my proud ego no longer lives. But the Messiah lives in me, and the life I now live in my body I live by the same trusting faithfulness that the Son of God had, who loved me and gave himself up for me. (CJB)

MEDITATION: I am dead to sin and sickness. Christ, the Messiah, lives in me. I share His resurrection life. The part of me that attracted sin and sickness lies dead and dormant. Christ Jesus in all His resurrection power is manifesting His life in me now. Every cell of my body is alive in Christ. I am dead to cancer; Christ's life is in me.

✞ ✞ ✞

1 Peter 2:24 and He Himself bore our sins in His body on the cross, so that we might die to sin and live to righteousness; for by His wounds you were healed.

24 who himself bore our sins in his body on the tree, in order that, being dead to sins, we may live to righteousness: by whose stripes ye have been healed. (Darby)

24 … by whose stripes, ye have been healed; (Rotherham)

24 who the sins of us himself carried up in the body of himself to the tree, that to the sins having died, to the righteousness we may live; of whom by the scars of him you were healed. (Wilson)

24 he himself cancel'd our sins by the crucifixion of his body, that we being set free from sin, might live in the service of virtue. It is by his bruises that you were healed: (Mace)

24 and took all our sins and upbore them in his body on the cross; that when dead to sin, in the righteousness of him we might live; for by his stripes you are healed (Etheridge)

24 … by whose wound ye were healed. (Whiston)

24 By his wounds you have been healed. (Goodspeed)

24 By His wounds yours have been healed. (Weymouth)

24 by Whose bruise ye were healed. (Worrell)

24 by whose stripes, [even] his, ye were healed. (Haweis)

24 His bruising was your healing. (Twentieth Century)

24 by whose stripes ye were healed, (Young)

24 He took our sins on himself, giving his body to be nailed on the tree, so that we, being dead to sin, might have a new life in righteousness, and by his wounds we have been made well. (Basic Bible)

MEDITATION: By Your wounds I was healed. It's a done deal. I'm not looking for healing. I was healed while You were on the cross. I accept Your sacrifice for me. Period.

✟ ✟ ✟

There's healing at the cross, and there's a trail from the cross to Pentecost. When the centurion stuck his spear into Christ Jesus' side, blood and water poured out. The blood was literal, it was His life; the water was literal and reminds us of His Spirit. The crucifixion leads to Pentecost. Without the cross there would be no Pentecostal outpouring of the Spirit. But, praise God, there is an outpouring. After ascending into heaven, the first act of the Savior was to sit at the right hand of the Father and from the throne release the Holy Spirit (Acts 2:33). Christ sent the Spirit to continue His healing ministry.

Chapter 14

God Heals You by His Spirit

I cannot emphasize the Spirit's role in healing strongly enough. First of all, it was the Holy Spirit who raised Jesus from the dead! The Spirit came into Him and gave Him life. That's what we all need, especially cancer sufferers. The Spirit is the opposite of death!

In addition, the Spirit is given by the Father to comfort and guide us. As you read in Part One, the dreams and "wake up thoughts" the Holy Spirit gave me were instrumental for my faith and direction. When I dreamed that I was running and playing basketball with small boys, I became elated. I was nearly ecstatic. I knew I was on the way to healing. Without the Spirit's encouragement, it would be hard to keep focusing faith and moving forward.

Come, Holy Spirit …

✞ ✞ ✞

Romans 8:11 But if the Spirit of Him who raised Jesus from the dead dwells in you, He who raised Christ Jesus from the dead will also give life to your mortal bodies through His Spirit who dwells in you.

11 But if the Spirit of him that raised up Jesus from the dead dwell in you, he that raised up Christ from the dead shall also quicken your mortal bodies by his Spirit that dwelleth in you. (KJV)

11 And if the Spirit of Him Who raised up Jesus from the dead dwells in you, [then] He Who raised up Christ Jesus from the dead will also restore to life your mortal (short-lived, perishable) bodies through His Spirit Who dwells in you. (AMP)

11 … he will, by that same Spirit, bring to your whole being new strength and vitality. (Phillips)

11 … With his Spirit living in you, your body will be as alive as Christ's! (MSG)

Romans 8:2 For the law of the Spirit of life in Christ Jesus has set you free from the law of sin and of death.

2 For the law of the Spirit of life in Christ Jesus hath made me free from the law of sin and death. (KJV)

2 For the law of the Spirit of life [which is] in Christ Jesus [the law of our new being] has freed me from the law of sin and of death. (AMP)

2 [For] Through [or In] Christ Jesus the law [principle; or power] of the Spirit that brings life set you free from the law [principle; or power] that brings sin and death. (EXP)

2 … because in Christ Jesus the law of the Spirit that brings life made you free. It made you free from the law that brings sin and death. (ERV)

2 … the Torah of the Spirit, which produces this life in union with Messiah Yeshua, has set me free from the "Torah" of sin and death. (CJB)

MEDITATION: The Spirit of God is dynamically alive in my body. He will never leave me nor forsake me. He is energizing my body, mind, and spirit today. He is life-giving and He is penetrating every cell of my body. He is a power, a force, an influence for life and health. He raised Jesus to life when He was dead and He is rejuvenating every cell in my mortal body today.

I can't lose! The law of the Spirit of life is lifting me up. His force is stronger than any force that's causing disease and bringing me down. God's Spirit is miraculously regenerating new tissues in my body. His creative power is forming new cells—nerves and muscles and anything else that's needed—in my physical body. He is creating life in me. He is creating life where there was no life.

The Holy Spirit of God is destroying every damaging cancer cell. He is using lethal force to zap every fungus, parasite, virus, or germ that is attacking me. Praise God!

✞ ✞ ✞

John 10:10 The thief comes only to steal and kill and destroy; I came that they may have life, and have it abundantly.

10 The thief cometh not, but for to steal, and to kill, and to destroy: I am come that they might have life, and that they might have it more abundantly. (KJV)

10 The thief comes only in order to steal and kill and destroy. I came that they may have and enjoy life, and have it in abundance (to the full, till it overflows). (AMP)

10 A thief comes [only] to steal and kill and destroy, but I came to give life [that they might have life]—life in all its fullness [abundance]. (EXP)

MEDITATION: Life! Life for now and eternity. By Your Spirit You are living in me. You have saved my life and now You are restoring my body. I will not die but live and declare the works of the Lord! Thank you for saving my life from the ravages of cancer.

✞ ✞ ✞

The devil tried to kill me. He is a robber, a thief, a killer, and is out to destroy me. Jesus is here to save, heal, restore, and give me abundance and energy. He is restoring my life right now. I will not die, but live and tell of the works of the Lord!

Chapter 15

God Heals You by Destroying the Devil's Works

Frankly, I can't always tell if the devil is doing something or if a disease is present due to natural causes. Discernment is not my greatest gift. What I have observed, however, is that the devil masquerades in natural events. That is to say, Satan causes some sicknesses that seem to all the world to be natural. He's a master at deception, which everyone who studies the Bible knows, but seldom recognizes in the matter of disease.

A teenage boy complained to me about headaches, which he said afflicted him several times each week. I didn't know what would cause such an unusual situation. I queried, "Is it stress?" and suggested he take a minute to massage the back of his neck. The thought came to me that perhaps the cause could be a demonic spirit masquerading as something very natural. I admitted to the boy I didn't know if this was an evil spirit or not, but suggested we do an experiment. With his permission, I proceeded to pray the blood of Jesus over him.

A few minutes later the young man announced, "My headache is gone!" A later inquiry told me that he had experienced no further headaches for a number of days.

Obviously, not every sickness is demonically induced. But some sicknesses are not solved until an evil spirit is dealt with.

☦ ☦ ☦

1 John 3:8 The Son of God appeared for this purpose, to destroy the works of the devil.

8 For this purpose the Son of God was manifested, that he might destroy the works of the devil. (KJV)

8 Now the Son of God came to the earth with the express purpose of liquidating the devil's activities. (Phillips)

8 The reason the Son of God was made manifest (visible) was to undo (destroy, loosen and dissolve) the works the devil [has done]. (AMP)

MEDITATION: I claim the finished work of Calvary. Lord, You said, "It is finished." Period. I believe it. I accept it. You came to destroy, undo, loosen, liquidate, and dissolve the devil's work. Sickness is not Your will for me. By faith, I destroy every cancer cell, every sickness, every germ, every harmful bacteria, fungus, and virus. By faith I may never be sick again because You have destroyed the devil's attempts to make me sick.

✝ ✝ ✝

Ephesians 6:10-12 Finally, be strong in the Lord and in the strength of His might. Put on the full armor of God, so that you will be able to stand firm against the schemes of the devil. For our struggle is not against flesh and blood, but against the rulers, against the powers, against the world forces of this darkness, against the spiritual forces of wickedness in the heavenly places.

11-12 Put on God's whole armor [the armor of a heavily armed soldier which God supplies], that you may be able successfully to stand up against [all] the strategies and the deceits of the devil. For we are not wrestling with flesh and blood [contending only with physical opponents], but against the despotisms, against the powers, against [the master spirits who are] the world rulers of this present darkness, against the spirit forces of wickedness in the heavenly (supernatural) sphere. (AMP)

10-12 Finally, be strengthened by the Lord and his powerful strength. Put on God's armor so that you can make a stand against the tricks of the devil. We aren't fighting against human enemies but against rulers, authorities, forces of cosmic darkness, and spiritual powers of evil in the heavens. (CEB)

11 … stand against the deceptive tactics of the Adversary. (CJB)

12 We are not fighting against humans. We are fighting against forces and authorities and against rulers of darkness and powers in the spiritual world. (CEV)

12 … fight against the devil's clever tricks. (ERV)

12 ... against supernatural powers and demon princes that slither in the darkness of this world, and against wicked spiritual armies that lurk about in heavenly places. (VOICE)

10-12 ... resist all the devil's methods of attack. For our fight is not against any physical enemy: it is against organizations and powers that are spiritual. We are up against the unseen power that controls this dark world, and spiritual agents from the very headquarters of evil. (PHILLIPS)

10-12 God is strong, and he wants you strong. So take everything the Master has set out for you, well-made weapons of the best materials. And put them to use so you will be able to stand up to everything the Devil throws your way. This is no afternoon athletic contest that we'll walk away from and forget about in a couple of hours. This is for keeps, a life-or-death fight to the finish against the Devil and all his angels. (MSG)

11-12 For we are not fighting against people made of flesh and blood, but against persons without bodies—the evil rulers of the unseen world, those mighty satanic beings and great evil princes of darkness who rule this world; and against huge numbers of wicked spirits in the spirit world. (TLB)

MEDITATION: Lord, You've opened my eyes to see how subtle these demonic influences are. Demons can make sickness seem natural. Sickness can masquerade as natural; in reality, it can be demonic.

You came to destroy and annul the works of the devil. I will not allow in my body or mind what you came to annul. What you came to destroy, I will not play with, give in to, or tolerate. What You destroy, by faith I destroy. I hate sickness. Right now, using all my power of focus and faith that I possess, I condemn these cancer cells and cast them out of my body, in Jesus' name! Done! In Jesus' name!

✞ ✞ ✞

James 4:7 Submit therefore to God. Resist the devil and he will flee from you.

7 Submit yourselves therefore to God. Resist the devil, and he will flee from you. (KJV)

7 Be subject, then, to God; stand up against the devil, and he will flee from you. (YLT)

7 So place yourselves under God's authority. Resist the devil, and he will run away from you. (GW)

7 Surrender to God! Resist the devil, and he will run from you. (CEV)

7 So submit yourselves to the one true God and fight against the devil and his schemes. If you do, he will run away in failure. (VOICE)

7 Therefore, submit to God. Moreover, take a stand against the Adversary, and he will flee from you. (CJB)

MEDITATION: I surrender myself to God. I am under Your authority. Whatever You say, I will obey. I am submitted to You. I am Your subject, Your servant. I have chosen to resist Satan. I am alert to dig in my heels against the devil and any disease he tries to bring on me. He is my adversary, not my friend. I stand against him with all my might and by the power of the Holy Spirit. I hate sin and all it does to me. I hate the devil and all his ways. He is the one who causes sickness and disease. I resist him now and expect all sickness to leave my body and mind. I am clean and forgiven. I expect all sickness and symptoms of disease to go away and stay away. Begone, Satan!

✞ ✞ ✞

Acts 10:38 You know of Jesus of Nazareth, how God anointed Him with the Holy Spirit and with power, and how He went about doing good and healing all who were oppressed by the devil, for God was with Him.

38 … healing all who were under the power of the devil … (NIV)

38 … healing all who were under the tyranny of the Devil … (HCSB)

38 … healing those injured by The Evil One … (Aramaic Bible in Plain English)

38 … curing all who were being continually oppressed by the Devil … (Weymouth)

MEDITATION: O Lord, I hate the devil. I hate all his works and all his ways. He no longer has any right to hurt me, oppress me, or make me sick in any way. Devil, I rebuke you now. Get away and stay away. You cannot oppress me, depress me, or suppress me. As stated in Colossians 1:12 and following, I am under the jurisdiction of the Lord Jesus Christ!

✞ ✞ ✞

Luke 10:17-19 … The seventy returned with joy, saying, "Lord, even the demons are subject to us in Your name." And He said to them, "I was watching Satan fall from heaven like lightning. Behold, I have given you authority to tread on serpents and scorpions, and over all the power of the enemy, and nothing will injure you."

17-19 … The seventy returned with joy, saying, Lord, even the demons are subject to us in Your name! And He said to them, I saw Satan falling like a lightning [flash] from heaven. Behold! I have given you authority and power to trample upon serpents and scorpions, and [physical and mental strength and ability] over all the power that the enemy [possesses]; and nothing shall in any way harm you. (AMP)

17-19 The 70 disciples came back very happy. They said, "Lord, even demons obey us when we use the power and authority of your name!" Jesus said to them, "I watched Satan fall from heaven like lightning. I have given you the authority to trample snakes and scorpions and to destroy the enemy's power. Nothing will hurt you." (GW)

17 … Lord, even the devils are subject unto us through thy name. (KJV)

18 … I beheld Satan as lightning fall from heaven. (KJV)

18 … Then he said to them, I saw him, Satana, when he fell as lightning from heaven. (Etheridge)

19 … Behold, I give unto you power to tread on serpents and scorpions, and over all the power of the enemy: and nothing shall by any means hurt you. (KJV)

19 … I have authoriz'd you to trample upon serpents and scorpions, and triumph over all the power of the enemy; so that nothing shall be capable of doing you any mischief. (MACE)

19 Lo! I empowered you to turn on serpents, and scorpions, and all the might of the enemy, and nothing shall hurt you. (Campbell)

MEDITATION: Jesus authorized me to cast out demons. I have the power and I'm using it. The devil is nothing but a fallen cherub. He has no power over me, none at all. He is defeated and I am victorious. I'm walking over him. Every demon and every demonic activity must go now, in Jesus' name!

I have repented of any inroads I've allowed. I've closed every door the Holy Spirit has shown me that allowed demonic activity. I'm clean and forgiven. The Lord rebuke you, Satan! Begone! I reject all sickness, numbness, pain, and disease. I speak God's life into my body right now, in Jesus' name.

☩ ☩ ☩

Colossians 1:12-14 … giving thanks to the Father, who has qualified us to share in the inheritance of the saints in Light. For He rescued us from the domain of darkness, and transferred us to the kingdom of His beloved Son, in whom we have redemption, the forgiveness of sins.

12 He has enabled you to share in the inheritance that belongs to his people (NLT)

12 … thanking the Father who makes us strong enough to take part in everything bright and beautiful that he has for us. (MSG)

13 … out of the authority [or jurisdiction, dominion] of darkness … (DLNT)

14 … who purchased our freedom … (NLT)

MEDITATION: Here I am, standing forever in the kingdom where Jesus rules. I'm a citizen of His kingdom. I was in the venue of darkness where Satan ruled. No more. The devil has nothing in me (John 14:30). I've been transferred; I have a new address and I'm living in the jurisdiction of Jesus. I'm under new authority, new management. Jesus is Lord over me now and forever, praise His name! I've been rescued by the blood, never to go back.

I won't worry whether or not I deserve this. Christ Jesus has qualified me for this new position. He made me fit by the blood of His cross. He has declared me fit, worthy by His merits. He has purchased me for Himself, enabled me, and made me eligible to claim my inheritance. I claim my healing now as part of my inheritance.

☩ ☩ ☩

Peter 5:8-9 Be of sober spirit, be on the alert. Your adversary, the devil, prowls around like a roaring lion, seeking someone to devour. But resist him, firm in your faith, knowing that the same experiences of suffering are being accomplished by your brethren who are in the world.

8-9 Be sober, be vigilant; because your adversary the devil, as a roaring lion, walketh about, seeking whom he may devour: Whom resist steadfast in the faith, knowing that the same afflictions are accomplished in your brethren that are in the world. (KJV)

8 Be well balanced (temperate, sober of mind), be vigilant and cautious at all times; for that enemy of yours, the devil, roams around like a lion roaring [in fierce hunger], seeking someone to seize upon and devour. (AMP)

9 Withstand him; be firm in faith [against his onset—rooted, established, strong, immovable, and determined], knowing that the same (identical) sufferings are appointed to your brotherhood (the whole body of Christians) throughout the world. (AMP)

MEDITATION: I will be sensitive, alert to any new forms of sickness trying to come on me. I will be vigilant at the first sign of a cold or infection because I know Satan tries to mimic sickness and make it seem so natural. I reject the onset of sickness. I take my stand against all sickness and symptoms in Jesus' name.

☦ ☦ ☦

One of my favorite songs goes like this: "God is so good, God is so good; He's so good to me." I used to sing it to our children when I was putting them in bed at night.

In some groups there is a famous shout "GOD IS GOOD!" The expected response should follow "ALL THE TIME!"

It's fun and the shouting declares God's nature—who He is and what He's like. It may surprise some who struggle to find healing, yet the truth is worth shouting from the housetops. Let the next chapter thunder the truth into your spirit: GOD IS GOOD, ALL THE TIME, AND IT'S HIS NATURE TO HEAL!

Chapter 16

God Heals—It's His Nature to Heal You

This excites me. It's God's nature to heal. During Bible studies we learn the attributes of God—omnipresent, omnipotent, omniscient, all loving, just, holy, merciful, and so on. Recently, through meditation on the word of God, I've discovered His very nature is to heal. It's who He is in the core of His being. Water wets, fish swim, birds fly, God heals.

An understanding of His nature as Healer comes by study of the Scriptures and revelation through the Holy Spirit. What a marvelous encouragement this is—to know Him as the One whose nature is to heal. Healing is not an add-on or side ministry. It's Him in totality. To know Him is to know Him as Healer. What a powerful doubt-crusher. If you're groping for spiritual healing, ask God to let you experience His true nature. An experience with His nature can transport you across the threshold into spiritual healing.

Absorb His presence, dwell in it, and enjoy it! This is healing for body, mind, and soul.

✝ ✝ ✝

Exodus 15:26 And He said, "If you will give earnest heed to the voice of the LORD your God, and do what is right in His sight, and give ear to His commandments, and keep all His statutes, I will put none of the diseases on you which I have put on the Egyptians; for I, the LORD, am your healer" [Yahweh-Rapha].

26 I am the Lord that healeth thee. (KJV)

26 for I the Lord am your physician. (Leeser)

26 For, I, am Yahweh, thy physician. (Rotherham)

26 for I, the Lord, make you immune to them [cancers]. (Smith-Goodspeed)

MEDITATION: Your nature is to heal. It's who You are. Fish swim, birds fly, You heal. It's that simple. "Healer" is who You are. "Healer" is Your inescapable core, Your character. Thank You for revealing Your true nature. To know You is to know You as Healer. I'm abiding in You and You're abiding in me. I'm being healed right now. Thank You.

Healing is not so much about my faith, my prayer, my need, or me. It's about You, Your nature, who You are.

I thank you Lord, that You are my total righteousness. I have no other. You have completely fulfilled God's laws and given me your perfect righteousness. I humbly hide myself in You. Now I take the healing from cancer and its side effects that You offer. You are my Healer. You are healing me right now. I'm in You and You're in me. Your name is "Healer." You are the same today as You were before. Your nature is in Your name. It is Your nature to heal and I'm receiving Your healing now.

✟ ✟ ✟

John 15:4-5 Abide in Me, and I in you. As the branch cannot bear fruit of itself unless it abides in the vine, so neither can you unless you abide in Me. I am the vine, you are the branches; he who abides in Me and I in him, he bears much fruit, for apart from Me you can do nothing.

4-5 Dwell in Me, and I will dwell in you. [Live in Me, and I will live in you.] Just as no branch can bear fruit of itself without abiding in (being vitally united to) the vine, neither can you bear fruit unless you abide in Me. I am the Vine; you are the branches. Whoever lives in Me and I in him bears much (abundant) fruit. However, apart from Me [cut off from vital union with Me] you can do nothing. (AMP)

4-5 You must go on growing in me and I will grow in you. For just as the branch cannot bear any fruit unless it shares the life of the vine, so you can produce nothing unless you go on growing in me. I am the vine itself, you are the branches. It is the man who shares my life and whose life I share who proves fruitful. For the plain fact is that apart from me you can do nothing at all. (Philips)

4-5 Live in me. Make your home in me just as I do in you. In the same way that a branch can't bear grapes by itself but only by being joined to the vine, you can't bear fruit unless you are joined with me. I am the Vine, you are the branches. When you're joined with me and I with you, the relation intimate and organic, the harvest is sure to be abundant. Separated, you can't produce a thing. (MSG)

MEDITATION: Lord Jesus, I'm living in You by faith, sticking really close. I don't want to leave You for a moment. Let my thoughts, both sleeping and awake, be from You. I'm growing in You and You're growing in me. Release me from any and all self-sufficiency.

I'm in union with You. I'm united to the healing vine. *Yahweh-Rapha* is in me and I'm in You. Your life and healing virtue are flowing into every cell of my body right now. I'm absorbing Your healing into my spirit, mind, and body right now. I'm like a sponge, taking in all of Your life into every organ of my body. My visible limbs are being healed, rejuvenated. The invisible organs inside my body are being transformed, healed, and made new by Your life in me.

You are *Yahweh-Rapha* and You will never leave me nor forsake me. I'm one with You, the healing vine and I'm taking in Your strength right now. To God be the glory!

✞ ✞ ✞

Deuteronomy 7:15 The LORD will remove from you all sickness; and He will not put on you any of the harmful diseases of Egypt which you have known, but He will lay them on all who hate you.

15 And the LORD will take away from thee all sickness, and will put none of the evil diseases of Egypt, which thou knowest, upon thee; but will lay them upon all them that hate thee. (KJV)

MEDITATION: You are the LORD. You are *Yahweh-Rapha*, the Lord our Healer. Healing is Your nature. It's who You are—the God who heals. And You are good. Disease is evil. Cancer is evil. The Lord has removed all cancer from my body. He got it all; no tumors, no cysts, no side effects remain. He is a faithful God. Not one of the good promises which He has made has failed. He is watching over His word to perform it. Praise God!

✞ ✞ ✞

Jeremiah 17:14 Heal me, O LORD, and I will be healed; Save me and I will be saved, For You are my praise.

14 Heal me, O Jehovah, and I am healed, Save me, and I am saved, for my praise art Thou. (Young)

MEDITATION: O Lord, I am healed by Your stripes. Your death at the cross dealt a death-blow to cancer. I am healthy today because of You. You are *Jehovah-Rapha*, the Lord our Healer. I will ever praise You for Your faithfulness. You are always true to Your name and Your word. You are not a man that You should lie. I trust You entirely. I'm getting to know You more. I know Your name. I even know how to pronounce it! You are *Jehovah-Rapha*. (Jeh-ho-vah-raw-faw) You always live up to Your name. Your name reveals Your nature. You never act apart from Your name! Thank you for healing me from cancer and its side effects.

NOTE: God is a happy God! *In Your presence is fullness of joy* (Psalm 16:11)! God's nature is joyous and playful. His very nature brings healing.

✞ ✞ ✞

Proverbs 17:22 A joyful heart is good medicine, but a broken spirit dries up the bones.

22 A merry heart doeth good like a medicine: but a broken spirit drieth the bones. (KJV)

22 Being cheerful keeps you healthy. (Good News)

22 A happy heart is a healing medicine … (Smith-Goodspeed)

22 A glad heart makes a healthy body … (Basic English)

22 A glad heart helps and heals … (Moffatt)

22 A glad heart is excellent medicine, a spirit depressed wastes the bones away. (Jerusalem)

22 A cheerful heart makes a quick recovery; it is crushed spirits that waste a man's frame. (Knox)

22 The best medicine is a cheerful heart … (Fenton)

22 A joyful heart worketh an excellent cure … (Rotherham)

22 … a broken spirit makes one sick. (Living Bible)

Nehemiah 8:10 … for the joy of the Lord is your strength. (NASB, KJV, HNV)

10 … for the joy of Jehovah is your strength (YLT, DBY)

MEDITATION: I'm strong today because You make me happy. Your joy is in me because You're in me and You are the happiest Man who ever lived (Hebrews 1:9). Your joyous nature is filling me with healing power.

Furthermore, You will never leave me nor forsake me. You're in me and I'm in You. Praise You! You are in my mind, my muscles, and my hormones. You are in my immune system making me so strong that I can overcome every cancer cell that tries to waste my body. Your joy is defeating discouragement and worry. Hallelujah, the more I praise You the stronger I get!

☦ ☦ ☦

Ho, ho, ho Hosanna;

Ha, ha, ha, Hallelujah;

He, he, he, He saved me;

I've got the joy of the Lord!

I've chosen to be happy. Cancer can't get me down. God is lifting me up! I have the best medicine and the best "Doctor." Cancer can't dominate me. Satan has no hold on me. I have a happy heart. God's medicine—God's word is healing me right now.[22]

While meditating on these Scriptures and sensing the healing power of Christ, I penned this poem.

I'm tromping on the pain,

Jesus' blood covers my shame;

In me stands the Man of fame—

Jehovah-Rapha is His Name.

MEDITATION: At Your Name, demons flee. At your Name, germs dissolve, sickness dissipates. At Your Name, tissues regenerate. Your Name stops pain. We are baptized into Your Name. Your Name is in us. We have the authority of Your Name. I rebuke all cancer and every other disease in my body right now in Jesus' Name.

☦ ☦ ☦

1 Corinthians 6:19-20 Or do you not know that your body is a temple of the Holy Spirit who is in you, whom you have from God, and that you are not your own? For you have been bought with a price: therefore glorify God in your body.

---

[22] (Cross Healed Hearts: Healing Scripture by Joyce Meyer, http://crosshealedhearts.blogspot.com/2010/07/healing-scripture-by-joyce-meyer.html_br (last accessed September 26, 2014).

19-20 What? Know ye not that your body is the temple of the Holy Ghost which is in you, which ye have of God, and ye are not your own? For ye are bought with a price: therefore glorify God in your body, and in your spirit, which are God's. (KJV)

MEDITATION: God Himself lives in me. My body is His temple. My body is the shrine of the Holy Spirit. I am His signpost, His advertisement. My body represents the Lord, the faithful healer. He is *Yahweh-Rapha*, the Lord our healer. He is in me, and He is healing me now. Cancer is incompatible with my body because I am a holy temple of the Spirit of God.

✟ ✟ ✟

Mark 5:25-34 And there was a woman who had had a flow of blood for twelve years,

And who had endured much suffering under [the hands of] many physicians and had spent all that she had, and was no better but instead grew worse.

She had heard the reports concerning Jesus, and she came up behind Him in the throng and touched His garment, For she kept saying, If I only touch His garments, I shall be restored to health.

And immediately her flow of blood was dried up at the source, and [suddenly] she felt in her body that she was healed of her [distressing] ailment.

And Jesus, recognizing in Himself that the power proceeding from Him had gone forth, turned around immediately in the crowd and said, Who touched My clothes?

And the disciples kept saying to Him, You see the crowd pressing hard around You from all sides, and You ask, Who touched Me?

Still He kept looking around to see her who had done it.

But the woman, knowing what had been done for her, though alarmed and frightened and trembling, fell down before Him and told Him the whole truth.

And He said to her, Daughter, your faith (your trust and confidence in Me, springing from faith in God) has restored you to health. Go in (into) peace and be continually healed and freed from your [distressing bodily] disease. (AMP)

28 ... for she kept saying, If I touch even his garments, I shall be made whole. (Wuest)

28 ... for she kept saying, 'If I can only touch his clothes, I shall get well.' (Williams)

28-30 "If I can put a finger on his robe, I can get well." The moment she did it, the flow of blood dried up. She could feel the change and knew her plague was over and done with. At the same moment, Jesus felt energy discharging from him. (MSG)

28-29 For she thought [margin, lit, was saying], "If I just touch His garments, I will get well." Immediately the flow of her blood was dried up; and she felt in her body that she was healed of her affliction. (NASB)

28-30 For she said, If I may touch but his clothes, I shall be whole. And straightway the fountain of her blood was dried up; and she felt in her body that she was healed of that plague. And Jesus, immediately knowing in himself that virtue had gone out of him ... (KJV)

MEDITATION: I'm desperate—I can't go on. I need complete restoration. I'm reaching out to You now. By faith, I'm touching You, I'm touching You, I'm touching You. You are my Savior, my Healer. You are *Yahweh-Rapha*, the Lord who heals. Your nature is overwhelming me. Your life and healing virtue are flowing into me right now. I'm being healed. Your virtue is coming into me. Your life-giving Spirit is moving throughout my body right now through faith. I have faith. Your faith is coming into me. Faith comes through You according to Acts 3:16 and Your faith is coming into me right now. I believe You and that assures me. Thank You, Lord Jesus.

✞ ✞ ✞

Psalm 42:11 Why art thou cast down, O my soul? And why art thou disquieted within me? Hope thou in God: for I shall yet praise him, who is the health of my countenance, and my God. (KJV)

11 ... for I will give thanks to him; [he is] the health of my countenance, and my God. (Brenton)

11 ... for I shall yet praise him, [who is] the health of my countenance, and my God. (Scrivener)

11 Wait thou for God, for yet shall I praise him, As the triumph of my presence and my God. (Rotherham)

11 … hope thou in God: for I shall yet praise him, who is the health of my countenance, and my God. (Webster)

11 Hope thou in God, for yit Y schal knouleche to hym; he is the helthe of my cheer, and my God. (Wycliffe, 1395)

11 Wait for God, for still I confess Him, The salvation of my countenance, and my God! (YLT)

11 Hope thou in God; for I shall yet thank him, the salvation of my countenance, and my God. (Leeser)

11 Fix my eyes on God—soon I'll be praising again. He puts a smile on my face. He's my God. (MSG)

MEDITATION: Yes, You are putting a smile on my face. I can stand straight and tall. I refuse to get discouraged or stay discouraged. No more frowns, no more dragging around. You are my health and my face shows it. I thank You and praise You. I worship You as the health of my countenance.

✞ ✞ ✞

Psalm 91:1-4 He who dwells in the shelter of the Most High Will abide in the shadow of the Almighty. I will say to the LORD, "My refuge and my fortress, My God, in whom I trust!" For it is He who delivers you from the snare of the trapper And from the deadly pestilence. He will cover you with His pinions, And under His wings you may seek refuge; His faithfulness is a shield and bulwark.

1-4 He that dwelleth in the secret place of the most High shall abide under the shadow of the Almighty. I will say of the LORD, He is my refuge and my fortress: my God; in him will I trust. Surely he shall deliver thee from the snare of the fowler, and from the noisome pestilence. He shall cover thee with his feathers, and under his wings shalt thou trust: his truth shall be thy shield and buckler. (KJV)

1-4 The praise of a canticle for David. He that dwelleth in the aid of the most High, shall abide under the protection of the God of Jacob. He shall say to the Lord: Thou art my protector, and my refuge: my God, in him will I trust. For he hath delivered me from the snare of the hunters: and from the sharp word. He will overshadow thee with his shoulders: and under his wings thou shalt trust. (Douay-Rheims)

3 ... and keep you safe from wasting disease [cancer]. (Basic English)

3 ... He will keep you safe from all hidden dangers and from all deadly disease. (Good News)

4 ... His faithful promises are your armor. (Living Bible)

4 You can go to him for protection. He will cover you like a bird spreading its wings over its babies. (ERV)

4 His truth is your shield and armor. (GW)

4 He will shield you with his wings! They will shelter you. His faithful promises are your armor. (TLB)

4 ... His truth [faithfulness] will be your shield and protection. (EXP)

MEDITATION: I'm hiding in the secret place of the Most High God. No evil shall befall me. None whatsoever! He is protecting me. I'm in His shadow. He is my Defender against all cancer, sickness, and disease. He's protecting me from the side effects of chemo treatments. I'm lodging in Christ; Christ is dwelling in me. I'm spending time with Him and He is Jehovah-Rapha, the Lord who heals me. Praise His Name!

I refuse to allow sin, sickness, or Satan in my life. I love righteousness and hate evil. Cancer is not from God. I refuse to let it grow in me. I cast out the spirit of cancer now. Begone, in Jesus' Name!

✞ ✞ ✞

Psalm 91:10-11 No evil will befall you, Nor will any plague come near your tent [dwelling]. For He will give His angels charge concerning you, To guard you in all your ways.

10-11 For he shall give his angels charge over thee, to keep thee in all thy ways. There shall no evil befall thee, neither shall any plague come nigh thy dwelling. (KJV)

10-11 No disaster will happen to you, no calamity will come near your tent; for he will order his angels to care for you and guard you wherever you go. (CJB)

There shall no evil befall you, nor any plague or calamity come near your tent. For He will give His angels [especial] charge over you to accompany and defend and preserve you in all your ways [of obedience and service]. (AMP)

10 So sickness will not approach you, contagion not enter your rest. (Fenton)

MEDITATION: Cancer cannot grow in my body. Cancer cannot spread in my body. Every cancer cell, every tumor, every cyst, must die, because You are my protection. You are my shield and my armor. I'm hidden under Your great wings of protection. No evil shall befall me; sickness cannot approach me. You are my Savior, my Safe-keeper.

✟ ✟ ✟

Psalm 91:14-16 Because he has loved Me, therefore I will deliver him; I will set him securely on high, because he has known My name. He will call upon Me, and I will answer him; I will be with him in trouble; I will rescue him and honor him. With a long life I will satisfy him And let him see My salvation.

14-16 Because he has set his love upon Me, therefore will I deliver him; I will set him on high, because he knows and understands My name [has a personal knowledge of My mercy, love, and kindness—trusts and relies on Me, knowing I will never forsake him, no, never]. He shall call upon Me, and I will answer him; I will be with him in trouble, I will deliver him and honor him. With long life will I satisfy him and show him My salvation. (AMP)

14-16 God says, "Because you are devoted to me, I'll rescue you. I'll protect you because you know my name. Whenever you cry out to me, I'll answer. I'll be with you in troubling times. I'll save you and glorify you. I'll fill you full with old age. I'll show you my salvation." (CEB)

14-16 "Because he clings to Me in love, I will rescue him from harm; I will set him above danger. Because he has known Me by name, He will call on Me, and I will answer. I'll be with him through hard times; I'll rescue him and grant him honor. I'll reward him with many good years on this earth and let him witness My salvation." (Voice)

14-16 Because he hath fixed his desire upon me, therefore will I release him: I will set him on high, because he knoweth my name. He will call on me, and I will answer him: with him will I be in distress; I will deliver him, and grant him honor. With length of days will I satisfy him, and I will let him see my salvation. (Leeser)

MEDITATION: I know Your Name! It's *Yahweh-Rapha*, the Lord our healer. Your name reveals Your nature. Your nature is in Your name. As I say Your name and meditate on it, Your nature is coming into me. Your name, Your nature, is "Healer." I desire to know Your name more fully. I want to feel Your name when I say it. Thank you for delivering me and honoring me. Thank you for healing me and granting me a long life. I daily enjoy Your healing Presence.

Lord, I deeply love You. I'm loving You more and more. The more I meditate on You, Your nature, and Your word, the more I love You. I have fixed my desire on You. I have chosen to obey You in every matter.

✞ ✞ ✞

Meditation on God's word is wonderful. Meditation brings enlightenment. Through meditation I found that healing is hidden in God's nature. Now I've discovered something even more amazing and it's the subject of the next chapter.

Chapter 17

God Heals—It's His Pleasure to Heal You

I have made a marvelous discovery. It came as a complete surprise. I've never heard anyone teach it or say it; nevertheless, it's hidden in the Scriptures. Some translations bring it out more than others. Here's a most wonderful surprise for anyone suffering and agonizing in pain: *It's God's pleasure to heal you!* Many times we struggle, doubt, and wrestle with God about healing. We just need to know God better. Continue and discover for yourself—it's God's pleasure to heal people! It's God's pleasure to heal you!

✞ ✞ ✞

Psalm 149:4 For the LORD takes pleasure in His people; He will beautify the afflicted ones with salvation [healing].

4 For the Lord is wel plesid in his puple; and he hath reisid [raised] mylde men in to heelthe [health]. (Wycliffe, 1395)

MEDITATION: Lord, Your pleasure is my healing. You delight in my healing and rightly so because You suffered and died for my wholeness. You don't want me to neglect what You suffered to give me. I will not grieve You by despising or ignoring Your gift to me.

Lord, beautify me now. Healing is part of Your great salvation. Beautify me with Your marvelous salvation as You delight in me. I am Your pleasure. It feels good to be in Your pleasure. I'm glad You take delight in me. You not only want to heal me, but it's Your pleasure to heal me. I praise You! My healing gives You pleasure. Hallelujah!

I want to experience Your pleasure. I want to feel Your love. I want to feel Your pleasure. I want to sense the pleasure You feel as You heal me. Thank You, I'm beginning to feel it now. It makes You happy to see me accept Your healing touch. Your delight makes me happy too. More, Lord, more!

✝ ✝ ✝

Luke 12:32 Do not be afraid, little flock, for your Father has chosen gladly to give you the kingdom.

32 Fear not, little flock; for it is your Father's good pleasure to give you the kingdom. (KJV, ASV)

32 Fear not, little flock, because your Father did delight to give you the reign. (YLT)

32 Fear not, little flock, for it has been the good pleasure of your Father to give you the kingdom. (DBY)

32 "So don't be afraid, little flock. For it gives your Father great happiness to give you the Kingdom." (NLT)

32 Be not afraid, the dear little flock! for your Father delighteth to give you the kingdom. (Rotherham)

32 Fear not, little flock; for your Father hath willed to give you the kingdom. (Etheridge)

Matthew 12:28 But if I cast out devils by the Spirit of God, then the kingdom of God is come unto you.

Matthew 9:35 Jesus was going through all the cities and villages, teaching in their synagogues and proclaiming the gospel of the kingdom, and healing every kind of disease and every kind of sickness.

35 And Jesus went about all the cities and villages, teaching in their synagogues, and preaching the gospel of the kingdom, and healing every sickness and every disease among the people. (KJV)

MEDITATION: O Lord, I praise You that Your kingdom includes healing and deliverance from demons! Your kingdom includes cure from cancer. I praise You that You have chosen gladly to give me Your kingdom! Thank You for showing me Your pleasure to give the kingdom. I'm feeling Your pleasure as You are healing me. You enjoy giving me the kingdom! You enjoy healing Your people! It's not a struggle for You; rather, healing is what You enjoy doing. Thank you—healing is Your delight for me. I receive Your healing now! Hallelujah!

✝ ✝ ✝

Hebrews 10:6-7 In whole burnt offerings and sacrifices for sins You have taken no pleasure. Then I said, "Behold … I have come to do Your will.

7 I have come to do what you want. CEV, ERV, GW, NCV, NOG

NOTE: The Greek term for "will" that is used in Hebrews 10:6 and 7 is *thelema*. It can be variously translated "will," "want", "choice," "desire" as in Ephesians 2:3, or "pleasure" as in the King James Version of Revelation 4:11.

It adds sweetness and motivation to exchange "pleasure" for "will" in a number of well-known bible passages. Instead of *Thy will be done*, we can legitimately translate, *Thy pleasure be done* (Mt 6:10). Instead of *My food is to do the will of Him who sent Me*, try *My food is to do the pleasure of Him who sent me* (John 4:34). "Will" is cold, "pleasure" is warm and inviting.

In the Hebrews 10 Scripture, I submit that "pleasure" is a preferred translation of the term *thelema* because it intentionally contrasts with the fact that the Lord takes "no pleasure" in the blood of animals which are sacrificed for Him.

Here is the point. Jesus affirmed, *Lo, I came to do Your pleasure*. Then He went out and healed many. He demonstrated the truth that healing is the pleasure of the One who sent Him. The one word *thelema* includes both will and pleasure.

Let's go further into the pleasure of God to heal. The Father had no pleasure in the sacrifices of goats or bulls. But Jesus came to do the pleasure of His father. *Lo, I have come to do Your pleasure*. Then He gave *His body on the cross … for by His wounds you were healed* (1 Pet 2:24). His death—God's pleasure—opened the healing door for all who enter in.

MEDITATION: Lord, I love Your pleasure. I'm grateful that You earnestly desire to heal me. As I come to You again and again for healing, I feel Your pleasure. I'm receiving Your healing right now. I love You ….

✞ ✞ ✞

Isaiah 53:10 But the LORD was pleased

To crush Him, He made Him sick (margin),

If He would render Himself as a guilt offering,

He will see His offspring,

He will prolong His days,

And the good pleasure of the LORD will prosper in His hand.

NOTE: The Hebrew word used in both the first and last phrases of Isaiah 53:10 is *chaphets*, which means "to delight in, take pleasure in, desire, be pleased with."

10 Yet it pleased the LORD to bruise him; he hath put him to grief: when thou shalt make his soul an offering for sin, he shall see his seed, he shall prolong his days, and the pleasure of the LORD shall prosper in his hand. (KJV)

10 And Jehovah hath delighted to bruise him, He hath made him sick. If his soul doth make an offering for guilt, He seeth seed—he prolongeth days, And the pleasure of Jehovah in his hand doth prosper. (YLT)

10 Yet the LORD was pleased to crush Him, He made Him sick (margin). When You make Him a restitution offering, He will see His seed, He will prolong His days, and by His hand, the LORD's pleasure will be accomplished. (HCSB)

10 Yet it was the will of the LORD to crush him; he has put him to grief (margin: he has made him sick); when his soul makes an offering for guilt, he shall see his offspring; he shall prolong his days; the will of the LORD shall prosper in his hand. (ESV)

10 Yet it was the will of the Lord to bruise Him; He has put Him to grief and made Him sick. When You and He make His life an offering for sin [and He has risen from the dead, in time to come], He shall see His [spiritual] offspring, He shall prolong His days, and the will and pleasure of the Lord shall prosper in His hand. (AMP)

10 Yet, Yahweh, purposed to bruise him, He laid on him sickness:—If his soul become an offering for guilt, He shall see a seed, He shall prolong his days,—And, the purpose of Yahweh, in his hand, shall prosper. (Rotherham)

MEDITATION: Father in heaven, You awe me. That You crushed Your Son, that You made Him sick is hard to swallow. And it was Your pleasure? Yes, it pleased You! And You did it for me! You bruised, crushed, and made Jesus sick for me! I'm moved with gratitude. For me! So I don't have to be sick or get sick. You loved me so much ….

The outcome? Your pleasure—my health and healing was accomplished. Yes, it was Your pleasure to heal me. I don't have to struggle to get healed. You already suffered enough for my healing. I don't have to push and pull, worry or cajole to receive what you so much desire to give me. Thank You for the gift of healing!

✞ ✞ ✞

Philippians 2:13 … for it is God who is at work in you, both to will and to work for His good pleasure.

13 For it is God which worketh in you both to will and to do of his good pleasure. (KJV)

13 for it is God who works in you both the willing and the working according to his good pleasure. (DBY)

13 … That energy is God's energy, an energy deep within you, God himself willing and working at what will give him the most pleasure. (MSG)

13 … to will and to work for His good pleasure and satisfaction and delight. (AMP)

MEDITATION: Healing is not only God's will for me; it is His pleasure. God is working in me and healing all cancer right now. He is showing me His pleasure to heal me. He is increasing my will to get healed. He is accomplishing total healing in me.

My healing is Your pleasure, O Lord. Nothing makes You happier than when I receive the benefits of Your suffering on the cross. I will not allow Your suffering to go for nothing. I will not waste Your stripes. I refuse to let Your agony go for nothing. By Your blood sacrifice, I am justified. By your sacrifice, I am made complete. Your sacrifice inspires my faith. By Your stripes I was healed. I accept Your healing—Your pleasure—right now.

✞ ✞ ✞

John 8:29 for I always do the things that are pleasing to Him.

29 for I do always those things that please him. (KJV, WEB)

NOTE: Jesus spent a major portion of His earthly ministry in healing and deliverance. He always did what pleased His Father. Since healing pleased the Father then, we can be certain healing pleases the Father now. Jesus Christ is the same yesterday, and today, and forever. Our healing pleases God!

MEDITATION: O Father, it was Your pleasure to heal the multitudes. It was Your pleasure to heal King Hezekiah. You were glad to heal the daughter of the Syro-Phoenician woman. You were happy to heal the centurion's slave. You delighted to heal the blind men of Jericho. It was Your pleasure to heal the leper who bowed before Jesus. And it is Your pleasure to heal me.

✟ ✟ ✟

Matthew 8:2-3 And a leper came to Him and bowed down before Him, and said, "Lord, if You are willing, You can make me clean." Jesus stretched out His hand and touched him, saying, "I am willing; be cleansed." And immediately his leprosy was cleansed.

2-3 Lord, if it is your pleasure, you have the power to make me clean. And he put his hand on him, saying, It is my pleasure; be clean. (Basic English)

2-3 A leper now came up and bowed low in front of him. 'Sir,' he said, 'if you want to, you can cure me.' Jesus stretched out his hand, touched him and said, 'Of course I want to! Be cured!' And his leprosy was cured at once. (Jerusalem)

2-3 "If you only choose, sir, you can cure me!" "I do choose! Be cured!" (Goodspeed)

2-3 "… if you have the will, you have the power to cleanse me." "… I have the will; be cleansed." (Wade)

2-3 "… Sir, if you really wanted to, you could heal me." "… I do want to. Be healed." (Jordan)

2-3 [A] leper came to him and worshiped him, saying, "Lord, if you want to, you can make me clean." And he stretched out his hand, and touched him, saying, "I want to. Be made clean." And immediately his leprosy was cleansed. (New Heart English Bible: Messianic Edition)

3 "… I am willing…" (Weymouth, Rotherham)

3 "… I am desiring it from all my heart. Be cleansed at once." (Wuest)

MEDITATION: O Lord, Your words are echoing in my spirit. "It is My pleasure, it is My pleasure, it is My pleasure." I know it's Your pleasure to heal me. You're not only willing to heal me, You are finding pleasure in healing me. I'm receiving Your pleasure as You are healing me. I feel Your pleasure as You are healing me.

Of course You want to heal me! After all, You paid the price for my healing at the cross. I will not let Your suffering for my healing go unused. I give You the pleasure of seeing the outcome of Your agony on the cross fulfilled in my body. You can be satisfied that it was worth it all. I accept my healing from cancer and every other disease right now. Thank You. Thank You. My cure is Your heart's desire fulfilled in me. Your pleasure is growing in me. I accept it.

✞ ✞ ✞

These verses anchor the wonderful reality: It's God's pleasure to heal. However, a question may linger in many regarding healing. "What is my responsibility?"

Chapter 18

God Heals You Through Repentance

Before there was sin, there was no sickness. When sin entered the world, disease and death followed. Sickness and sin are related, but not on a one-to-one basis. That is, one sin does not equal one sickness. One great sin does not equal one great sickness. The relationship of sin with disease can be stated in this way: When humanity fell into sin through Adam, humankind became subject to disease and death.

Sin has consequences. We can't deny the relationship of iniquity and disease. Jesus told the man at the Pool of Bethesda, *Behold, you have become well; do not sin anymore, so that nothing worse may befall you* (John 5:32). How else do we know sin has consequences? Deuteronomy chapter 28 makes the matter crystal clear. Read it if you have doubts.

But take heart. Forgiveness also has consequences! Here's the good news that brings healing and restores health. When sin is dealt with, healing can follow. Jesus addressed the paralyzed man before He healed him, *"Son, your sins are forgiven"* (Mark 2:5).

I once prayed for a man with severe deafness. Nothing happened. Then via a word of knowledge, I realized the man needed to forgive. It turned out the fellow had been imprisoned during World War II. A cruel prison guard had tortured him unmercifully. After the hearing-impaired man repented of hatred and forgave his torturer, I cast out the spirit of deafness. His hearing was immediately restored to normal.

Sometimes a father's sin can cause a person to become sick. Physicians know this. That's one reason doctors require a patient to fill out a medical history sheet before treatment. Past sins and generational curses must often be dealt with before receiving healing.

Sometimes physical and emotional healings burst upon a person after dealing with sin and the sin nature. However, sin is not always the cause of sickness. *And His disciples asked Him, "Rabbi, who sinned, this man or his parents, that he would be born blind?" Jesus answered, "It was neither that this man sinned, nor his parents; but it was so that the works of God might be displayed in him"* (John 9:2-3).

Truth bears repeating. Disease and death are in the world today affecting all humanity as a result of Adam's sin, yet sin and sickness are not always directly related in each individual. Personal sin may cause personal sickness, but we are not necessarily sick because of some sin we have committed.

If we know of sin in our life, we need to repent, ask forgiveness, make restitution if required, then come to Christ for healing.

We don't always know if sin is blocking our healing. Maybe it is or maybe not. How can we find out? The key is to ask the Holy Spirit. He is given by God the Father to help us. The Holy Spirit will gently convict us if we need repentance. He will also keep us from condemning ourselves for things already forgiven.

What should we do whenever we become aware of sin in our life? Good question. Merely trying hard doesn't always solve the problem. We need a Savior. Romans Chapter 6 goes to the heart of the sin issue and has served as the master sin-slayer in my life.

✞ ✞ ✞

Romans 6:6 … knowing this, that our old self was crucified with Him, in order that our body of sin might be done away with, so that we would no longer be slaves to sin

6 For we know that our old self was crucified with Him in order that sin's dominion over the body may be abolished, so that we may no longer be enslaved to sin (HCSB)

6 We know that our old (unrenewed) self was nailed to the cross with Him in order that [our] body [which is the instrument] of sin might be made ineffective and inactive for evil, that we might no longer be the slaves of sin. (AMP)

6 We know that the persons we used to be were nailed to the cross with Jesus. This was done, so that our sinful bodies would no longer be the slaves of sin. (CEV)

6 We know that our old sinful selves were crucified with Christ so that sin might lose its power in our lives. We are no longer slaves to sin. (NLT)

MEDITATION: O Lord, I have dealt with the sin issue. I have repented of all known sin. I have brought my sin nature to the cross. I was co-crucified with Christ. When He died to sin, I died with Him, by faith. When He was buried, I was buried with Him. I am a dead man to sin. I have been crucified with Christ. When He was raised, I was co-raised with Him, by faith. It is no longer I who live; now it is Christ who lives in me.

✞ ✞ ✞

James 5:14-16 Is anyone among you sick? Then he must call for the elders of the church and they are to pray over him, anointing him with oil in the name of the Lord; and the prayer offered in faith will restore the one who is sick, and the Lord will raise him up, and if he has committed sins, they will be forgiven him. Therefore, confess your sins to one another, and pray for one another so that you may be healed. The effective prayer of a righteous man can accomplish much.

14-16 Is any sick among you? Let him call for the elders of the church; and let them pray over him, anointing him with oil in the name of the Lord: And the prayer of faith shall save the sick, and the Lord shall raise him up; and if he have committed sins, they shall be forgiven him. Confess your faults one to another, and pray one for another, that ye may be healed. The effectual fervent prayer of a righteous man availeth much. (KJV)

14-16 Is any infirm among you? Let him call for the elders of the assembly, and let them pray over him, having anointed him with oil, in the name of the Lord, and the prayer of the faith shall save the distressed one, and the Lord shall raise him up, and if sins he may have committed, they shall be forgiven to him. Be confessing to one another the trespasses, and be praying for one another, that ye may be healed; very strong is a working supplication of a righteous man (YLT)

14-16 Are any of you sick? You should call for the elders of the church to come and pray over you, anointing you with oil in the name of the Lord. Such a prayer offered in faith will heal the sick, and the Lord will make you well. And if you have committed any sins, you will be forgiven. Confess your sins to each other and pray for each other so that you may be healed. The earnest prayer of a righteous person has great power and produces wonderful results. (NLT)

MEDITATION: Lord, I have confessed all known sin and made things right with the people against whom I have sinned. I am forgiven. I am clean by the blood of Your cross. I have been healed by the supplication of faith. The prayer of faith was spoken over me. I am healed. Nothing is stopping Your virtue from flowing into me. I am healed by Your stripes and by Your word. I receive complete healing. I'm not trying to get healing. I am healed and I'm acting like it.

✞ ✞ ✞

Perhaps the most common questions about spiritual healing regard faith. "Do I have enough faith?" "If I'm not yet better, is it because I don't have enough faith?" "What is the role of faith when it comes to healing?"

Chapter 19

God Heals You Through Faith

God's word is like the medicine we get at the pharmacy. Take the prescription according to directions; the medicine of God's word does the rest. As the Living Word and the written word find their place in us, faith happens. As we said earlier, "Listen, instead of wondering whether you have enough faith to be healed, just take the medicine. The faith will be there when you need it." It's a wonderful fact: faith comes through Jesus to the open heart.

Faith is the subject of the next meditation. And here's a reminder: all of Part Three is not for reading—it's for meditation and confession. It's for the power of God and the life of Jesus to come into your spirit and body and mind. It's for your healing. Anyone who skims, or merely reads this chapter, may find a blessing, but most likely will not receive the power.

Faith comes by hearing, and hearing by the word of Christ (Romans 10:17). Please note that the most ancient New Testament manuscripts do not say "word of God," but rather, "word of Christ." Meditation can turn the *logos* word into a *rhema* word. Mulling prayerfully over the written word is able to transform it into the spoken word of Christ. Spending time with a particular truth can transform the promised word into a personal word. We need to meditate until the living Christ imparts His word into our spirit. That's the power that heals.

✝ ✝ ✝

Acts 3:16 And on the basis of faith in His name, it is the name of Jesus which has strengthened this man whom you see and know; and the faith which comes through Him has given him this perfect health in the presence of you all.

16 And his name through faith in his name hath made this man strong, whom ye see and know: yea, the faith which is by him hath given him this perfect soundness in the presence of you all. (KJV)

16 And His name, through faith in His name, has made this man strong, whom you see and know. Yes, the faith which comes through Him has given him this perfect soundness in the presence of you all. (NKJV)

16 By faith in His name, His name has made this man strong, whom you see and know. So the faith that comes through Him has given him this perfect health in front of all of you. (HCSB)

MEDITATION: Faith comes through Jesus. I don't have to work it up. As I'm meditating on Your name, faith is coming from You into me. Faith is coming into my spirit right now. I'm in You and You're in me. Your faith, Yahweh-Rapha, is growing in me, getting stronger as I meditate on Your name.

At the name of Jesus every knee shall bow. Every cancer-causing virus and parasite must bow before the name of Jesus. I speak Your name, "Jesus," over my entire body right now.

Your name, Jesus—Savior, Healer, Deliverer—powers my healing. All that You are is in Your name. All of Your healing virtue is in Your name. Your name reflects Your nature. *Your nature is healing.* Your name through faith in Your name is strengthening me and giving me perfect health in every part of my body right now. Your name is greater than cancer: cancer has a little "c." Christ has a capital "C." Praise Your name!

✞ ✞ ✞

Mark 11:22 Have faith in God (NASB, KJV, NKJV, NIV, HCSB, DBY, ESV)

22 Have faith of God (YLT)

MEDITATION: Jesus, this is Your command. You are giving an imperative, not a suggestion. I cannot fulfill your command in my own strength because doubts pop up in my head. I can only fulfil this command by the power of the Holy Spirit. You never intended your children to fulfill your commands in our own strength. You always intended us to fulfill your commands by the power of the Holy Spirit.

Come, Holy Spirit, complete this command in me now. I receive the faith of God. I have faith in God through the Spirit. I have faith in God. I have faith in God by Your Spirit. God's faith is in me now. Seal Your faith which is in me.

✞ ✞ ✞

Mark 11:23-24 Truly I say to you, whoever says to this mountain, 'Be taken up and cast into the sea,' and does not doubt in his heart, but believes that what he says is going to happen, it will be granted him. Therefore, I say to you, all things for which you pray and ask, believe that you have received them, and they will be granted you.

23-24 For verily I say unto you, That whosoever shall say unto this mountain, Be thou removed, and be thou cast into the sea; and shall not doubt in his heart, but shall believe that those things which he saith shall come to pass; he shall have whatsoever he saith. Therefore I say unto you, What things soever ye desire, when ye pray, believe that ye receive them, and ye shall have them. (KJV)

MEDITATION: I'm telling you, "Cancer, get out of my body now. You cannot stay. Be gone. Be removed. On the basis of Jesus' word, I command you to go. Depart now and forever in Jesus Name."

"Body, be made whole." God's word trumps my feeling. What He says happens. I trust God and His word. I believe I have received healing. I'm feeding my faith and doubting my doubts. Healing is being manifested in my body right now. To God be the glory!

✞ ✞ ✞

Matthew 19:26 With people this is impossible, but with God all things are possible.

26 With men this is impossible; but with God all things are possible. (KJV)

26 "With humans, this is impossible. But with God, all things are possible." (DLNY)

Matthew 21:21 And Jesus answered and said to them, "Truly I say to you, if you have faith and do not doubt, you will not only do what was done to the fig tree, but even if you say to this mountain, 'Be taken up and cast into the sea,' it will happen.

21 Jesus responded, "I assure you that if you have faith and don't doubt, you will not only do what was done to the fig tree. You will even say to this mountain, 'Be lifted up and thrown into the lake.' And it will happen. CEB

21 Yeshua answered them, "Yes! I tell you, if you have trust and don't doubt, you will not only do what was done to this fig tree; but even if you say to this mountain, 'Go and throw yourself into the sea!' it will be done. CJB

21 Jesus answered, "The truth is, if you have faith and no doubts, you will be able to do the same as I did to this tree. And you will be able to do more. You will be able to say to this mountain, 'Go, mountain, fall into the sea.' And if you have faith, it will happen. ERV

21 But Jesus was matter-of-fact: "Yes—and if you embrace this kingdom life and don't doubt God, you'll not only do minor feats like I did to the fig tree, but also triumph over huge obstacles. This mountain, for instance, you'll tell, 'Go jump in the lake,' and it will jump. Absolutely everything, ranging from small to large, as you make it a part of your believing prayer, gets included as you lay hold of God." MSG

MEDITATION: I have faith. Your faith is in me. Cancer, go! Pain, go! Numbness, go! Thank You, Lord.

✞ ✞ ✞

Mark 9:23 And Jesus said to him, "'If You can?' All things are possible to him who believes."

23 Jesus said unto him, If thou canst believe, all things are possible to him that believeth. (KJV)

23 If I can?" Jesus asked. "Anything is possible if you have faith." (TLB)

23 "If you can do anything!" retorted Jesus. "Everything is possible to the man who believes." (PHILLIPS)

23 … "Why did you say 'if you can'? All things are possible for the one who believes." (ERV)

MEDITATION: I'm not questioning You. I believe You. You can do anything. I trust You today for my healing. Thank You, Lord Jesus.

✞ ✞ ✞

Mark 16:17-18 These signs [or attesting miracles] will accompany those who have believed: in My name they will cast out demons, they will speak with new tongues; they will pick up serpents, and if they drink any deadly poison, it will not hurt them; they will lay hands on the sick, and they will recover.

17-18 And these signs will accompany those who do trust: in my name they will drive out demons, speak with new tongues, not be injured if they handle snakes or drink poison, and heal the sick by laying hands on them. (CJB)

17 ... for those who believe, these miracles will follow ... (Moffatt)

17 ... These are the visible demonstrations of the action of God which will accompany the life of those who believe. (Barclay)

MEDITATION: Lord, I'm believing You for the demonstration of Your power in my life and in the lives of others. I'm believing You today for signs and wonders, miracles and healings. You said it, and I'm trusting You for it today through my prayers and the laying on of my hands.

I'm expecting supernatural actions from You, whether immediate or gradual. You are the same today as You were on earth. I'm taking advantage of opportunities to move in the supernatural realm.

☦ ☦ ☦

Matthew 15:26 And He answered and said, "It is not good to take the children's bread and throw it to the dogs." But she said, "Yes, Lord; but even the dogs feed on the crumbs which fall from their masters' table." Then Jesus said to her, "O woman, your faith is great; it shall be done for you as you wish." And her daughter was healed at once.

MEDITATION: O Lord, thank you for special favor and provision for Your children. Thank you that healing is our food, our bread, our daily staple. Healing is our bread of life, what You as a good Father gladly give to Your children. We expect it. Healing belongs to us. Healing belongs to the church. Healing is the bread and butter of the church. Healing is my food. You are feeding me with the bread of healing. I'm feasting on it now. Your food is healing me now.

☦ ☦ ☦

Proverbs 12:18 There is one who speaks rashly like the thrusts of a sword, But the tongue of the wise brings healing.

18 There is that speaketh like the piercings of a sword: but the tongue of the wise is health. (KJV)

18 There are some whose uncontrolled talk is like the wounds of a sword, but the tongue of the wise makes one well again. (Basic English)

MEDITATION: No longer am I cutting myself down and holding back my healing by telling people, "I have cancer." No way! Rather, I say, "God is healing me. I'm getting stronger!" Or, "I have some cancer symptoms and I'm believing God to remove them."

Lord, You've given me wisdom about what to say to people. It's never wrong to say what You say in Your word. Your word says, *By His wounds you were healed* (1 Peter 2:24). Now I say, "By Your wounds I was healed." My mouth is making me well. Thank you, Lord Jesus! *Death and life are in the power of the tongue* (Proverbs 18:21). I choose to control my tongue; I choose to speak life to my own body.

✞ ✞ ✞

Psalm 97:10 Hate evil, you who love the LORD, Who preserves the souls of His godly ones; He delivers them from the hand of the wicked.

10 Ye that love the LORD, hate evil: he preserveth the souls of his saints; he delivereth them out of the hand of the wicked. (KJV)

10 Ye lovers of Yahweh! Be haters of wrong – He preserveth the lives of his men … (Rotherham)

Hebrews 1:9 You [Jesus] have loved righteousness and hated lawlessness; therefore God, Your God, has anointed You with the oil of gladness above Your companions.

9 Thou hast loved righteousness, and hated iniquity; therefore God, even thy God, hath anointed thee with the oil of gladness above thy fellows. (KJV)

9 Thou didst love righteousness, and thou didst hate lawlessness; on account of this anointed thee the God of thee, oil of extreme joy beyond the associates of thee. (Benjamin Wilson)

9 Thou hast loved righteousness, and hast hated iniquity; therefore Aloha thy God hath anointed thee with the oil of exultation more (abundantly) than thy fellows. (Etheridge)

9 You have loved right and hated wrong! That is why God, your God, has anointed you with exhilarating oil beyond all your comrades. (Goodspeed)

Proverbs 18:21 Death and life are in the power of the tongue, and those who love it will eat its fruit.

21 Death and life are in the power of the tongue: and they that love it shall eat the fruit thereof. (KJV)

21 The tongue can bring death or life. (NLT)

MEDITATION: OK, Lord, I get the picture. What I say about myself and about sickness is supremely important. I want that exhilarating happiness that You have. You are happier than anyone around You, and I want to be like You!

I love You and I hate evil. I love You very much and I hate cancer and all it has done to my body. I hate it, I hate it, I hate it! I reject all tumors and cysts. I reject all bacteria, fungi, parasites, viruses, germs, and anything else that causes cancer. I hate everything bad for my body and soul. By faith, I'm getting rid of those things now.

I love You; I love righteousness. I give You credit for making me whole. I honor You. I eschew drawing attention to myself for being sick. You're my Healer and I praise You now! You have delivered me from the devil and all his works. I will not give in to evil.

Death to cancer! Death to pain! Death to paralysis! Death to numbness! Death to fear and to every evil thing associated with cancer. I speak life to my body and mind. You are my Life-giver. I will not die, but live, and tell of the works of the LORD (Psalm 118:17). Hallelujah!

✝ ✝ ✝

Psalm 103:2-3 Bless the Lord, O my soul, And forget none of His benefits; Who pardons all your iniquities, Who heals all your diseases;

2-3 Let all that I am praise the LORD; may I never forget the good things He does for me. He forgives all my sins and heals all my diseases. (NLT)

2-3 Bless (affectionately, gratefully praise) the Lord, O my soul, and forget not [one of] all His benefits—Who forgives [every one of] all your iniquities, Who heals [each one of] all your diseases, (AMP)

MEDITATION: O Lord, I aim to make You happy. It's Your pleasure to heal me. Your Name is Yahweh-Rapha (Jehovah-Rapha) and You are living up to Your sacred name. You are fulfilled when I am healed.

I praise You for each and every one of Your benefits. Thank You for including healing in the atonement. You have forgiven me all my sins and failures. All my disobedience and rebellion was nailed to the cross with You. I am complete in You. You pardoned all my resistance. You cured all my cancer. No disease can stay in my body for You have healed all my sicknesses.

✞ ✞ ✞

Have you been waiting for healing for a long time? Do you want someone to take a stand with you in faith? You may want to contact the Ministry Team at The Church of the Living Water.

We have a man in our church with a healing ministry. Bernie says the thing that gives him confidence to pray for people is the covenant. What is the covenant and how does it work?

Chapter 20

God Heals You Through His Covenant

Covenant is not a commonly used word today. Because of its infrequent usage, I need to explain the meaning and significance of the term.

Covenant is not a contract; it's much more. The words "guarantee" and "warranty" come closer to the meaning of covenant, but still fall short of the strength and significance of the term. A covenant is not merely an agreement between two parties.

The term "covenant" means an arrangement made by one party which the other party involved can accept or reject, but cannot alter. Three biblical examples of covenant demonstrate the strength of the term and show the power of a covenant for all who desire healing of body and soul.

God made a covenant with Abraham (Genesis 15). The biblical term is actually "cut" a covenant, referring to the practice of butchering animals and passing between the halves to show what will happen to anyone who breaks the arrangement once it has been ratified. This is especially striking in the case of God's covenant with Abraham. The flaming torch representing God Himself passed through the dismembered heifer, goat, and ram. Wow! God was saying in effect, "If I break this promise which I've just made, this will happen to Me!"

Ruth made a covenant with Naomi and sealed her vow with these memorable words. "*Where you die, I will die, and there I will be buried. Thus may the Lord do to me, and worse, if anything but death parts you and me*" (Ruth 1:17). I don't know how Ruth gestured when she said "thus," but I speculate she drew her hand like a sword and swept it across her jugular to act out the slitting of her throat.

Joshua covenanted with the deceptive Gibeonites to let them live (Joshua 9). The year was about 1400 BC. From that time on, the Israelites protected and defended the people of Gibeon, even though they didn't want to. They had to fight for the pagan Gibeonites and risk their lives for them because of the oath which Joshua and the leaders had made. The covenant, once made, was binding. A problem arose, however, during the reign of King Saul (about 1040-1000 BC). Saul, in his zeal to rid the heathen from the land, killed some of the Gibeonite descendants. Nothing happened until shortly before the year 960 BC toward the end of King David's reign. Suddenly, and for no apparent reason, a famine broke out in Israel that lasted for three years. David finally cried out to God to find the cause of the famine. The cause? Saul broke the covenant Israel had made with Gibeon (2 Samuel 21:1-2).

These events show the nearly unimaginable strength of covenant in God's eyes. Consider these facts. One, God bound Himself to honor the covenant. His covenant with Abraham still operates today (Galatians 3:6-29). Two, the covenant Joshua made included no "sunset clause"; it was valid and effectual at least 440 years. Three, God supernaturally worked in behalf of these covenants, even though the agreement Joshua made with the Gibeonites was based on deception.

> Jesus Christ is Himself the sum and substance of the covenant, and one of its gifts. He is the property of every believer. Believer, can you estimate what you have gotten in Christ? Our blessed Jesus, as God, is omniscient, omnipresent, and omnipotent. Has He power? That power is yours to support and strengthen you, to overcome your enemies, and to preserve you even to the end. Has He love? Well, there is not a drop of love in His heart which is not yours; you may dive into the immense ocean of His love, and you may say of it all, "It is mine." ... [sic] All that He has as perfect man is yours. "In Him dwells all the fullness of the Godhead bodily." Consider that word, "God" and its infinity, and then meditate upon "perfect man" and all His beauty; for all that Christ, as God and man, ever had, or can have, is yours. As perfect man the Father's delight was upon Him. All that Christ did is yours.[23]

Another word for covenant is "testament." We can speak either of the New Testament or the New Covenant. The content of the New Covenant is

---

[23] Charles Haddon Spurgeon from the Revival Study Bible, © 2010 by Armour Publishing Pte Ltd.

all that's contained in the New Testament. Does the New Testament in our Bible include healing? Most certainly!

How does this affect our healing today? God is honor-bound to bring healing to His people of faith. Healing is not based on human goodness; instead, it is guaranteed by God's covenantal word.

✞ ✞ ✞

Luke 22:20 And in the same way He took the cup after they had eaten, saying, "This cup which is poured out for you is the new covenant in My blood."

20 In the same way, after supper [they had eaten], Jesus took the cup and said, "This cup [or This cup that is poured out…] is the new agreement [covenant; a binding relationship between God and his people; Jer. 31:31–34] that begins with [that is established by; or that is sealed with; in] my blood …" (EXP)

20 And in like manner, He took the cup after supper, saying, This cup is the new testament or covenant [ratified] in My blood, which is shed (poured out) for you. (AMP)

20 After the meal he took another cup of wine in his hands. Then he said, "This is my blood. It is poured out for you, and with it God makes his new agreement." (CEV)

20 After supper he gave them another glass of wine, saying, "This wine is the token of God's new agreement to save you—an agreement sealed with the blood I shall pour out to purchase back your souls." (TLB)

20 In the same way He also took the cup after supper and said, "This cup is the new covenant established by My blood; it is shed for you." (HCSB)

Hebrews 7:22 so much the more also Jesus has become the guarantee of a better covenant.

22 By so much was Jesus made a surety of a better testament. (KJV)

22 In keeping with [the oath's greater strength and force], Jesus has become the Guarantee of a better (stronger) agreement [a more excellent and more advantageous covenant]. (AMP)

22 This makes Jesus the guarantee of a far better way between us and God—one that really works! A new covenant. (MSG)

22 in so much Jesus is made [better] promiser of the better testament. (WYC)

22 So we can see that Jesus has become the guarantee of a new and better covenant. (VOICE)

MEDITATION: Now I know my healing is sure. It's part of the covenant sealed in blood. You are the Guarantee of my health. No evil will befall me nor even come close to my family or me. You Yourself are my surety, my security, my assurance of health and healing. I praise You! I'm resting in the assurance that You are the "Promiser" of the covenant.

I thank You that we have a better covenant than the old one with Moses. Now we have an unconditional covenant, an agreement signed and sealed with Your own precious blood. You are the Guarantee of my healing. I praise You!

✞ ✞ ✞

Hebrews 8:10-11 For this is the covenant that I will make with the house of Israel after those days, says the Lord: I will put My laws into their minds, and I will write them on their hearts. And I will be their God, and they shall be my people. And they shall not teach everyone his fellow citizen, and everyone his brother, saying, 'Know the Lord,' for all will know Me, from the least to the greatest of them.

MEDITATION: O Lord, Thank You for the New Covenant that Jesus has mediated for us. Your Torah, Your teachings are inside of us and they are powerful.

I know You, just as the prophet Jeremiah promised! I know Your name. You are Jehovah-Rapha, the Lord our Healer. I know Your nature—the healing God. It's Your nature to heal. I know that You are always true to Your nature. I know You have chosen to heal us and that it is Your pleasure to heal. Thank You. I accept Your healing now.

O Lord, You are the Mediator of the New Covenant. Yet You are more than the Mediator, You are the Binding Covenant Yourself. You, in Your blood and in Your person, are the bond between the Father and me. You are the "Binder" that holds us together. You Yourself are the assurance of every promise of God. You are my Covenant Healer.

✞ ✞ ✞

Isaiah 49:8 Thus says the LORD, "In a favorable time I have answered You, And in a day of salvation I have helped You; And I will keep You and give You for a covenant of the people, To restore the land, to make them inherit the desolate heritages;

8 Thus saith the LORD, In an acceptable time have I heard thee, and in a day of salvation have I helped thee: and I will preserve thee, and give thee for a covenant of the people … (KJV)

8 Thus says the Lord, In an acceptable and favorable time I have heard and answered you, and in a day of salvation I have helped you; and I will preserve you and give you for a covenant to the people, to raise up and establish the land [from its present state of ruin] and to apportion and cause them to inherit the desolate [moral wastes of heathenism, their] heritages, (AMPC)

8 The LORD said: At the right time, I answered you; on a day of salvation, I helped you. I have guarded you, and given you as a covenant to the people … (CEB)

8 Eternal One: When the time was right, I answered you; on the day you were delivered, I was your help. I will watch over you, and give you as a promise, a binding covenant to the people. (VOICE)

MEDITATION: Jesus Christ, You are Yourself the sum and substance of the New and Everlasting Covenant. When You said, "This is My blood of the covenant," You gave Yourself as the covenant. I take You in. I am absorbing You like a sponge. All that You are, I receive. All that You have, I receive. All that You have ever done, I receive. All that You will do, I accept.

You are the covenant God in all Your supremacy. All Your credits You have given to me. All Your healing powers are now mine and at my disposal. All my debits, doubts, weakness and failures I give to You. You are mine and I am Yours.

I lay claim today to my spiritual and physical inheritance. You have qualified me to take my full inheritance. The promises I have not claimed in the past, I claim today. I take full healing into my mind, body, nerves, and cells. Where chemotherapy ruined healthy tissues, I claim restoration. What has been wasted, unclaimed, destroyed, or gone to ruin, I claim today. You have re-assigned to me complete health. I am complete in You.

You are the covenant Man, in all Your beauty. All that You are as complete Man, I accept by faith as my own. In You dwells all the fullness of

Godhead in bodily form. I accept complete restoration of my body, mind and soul. I accept Your infinite love. I accept the fullness of Your joy. I accept YOU as the Person of the covenant.

✞ ✞ ✞

Hebrews 13:20 Now the God of peace, who brought up from the dead the great Shepherd of the sheep through the blood of the eternal covenant, even Jesus our Lord …

20 Now may the God of peace [Who is the Author and the Giver of peace], Who brought again from among the dead our Lord Jesus, that great Shepherd of the sheep, by the blood [that sealed, ratified] the everlasting agreement (covenant, testament) (AMP)

20 He raised him because Jesus sacrificed his blood to begin the new agreement that never ends. (ERV)

20 … as the result of his blood, by which the eternal covenant is sealed. (GNT)

20 … back from the dead through the blood of the new everlasting covenant (VOICE)

20 … through the blood of the everlasting covenant (KJV)

20 … by an everlasting agreement between God and you, signed with his blood (TLB)

MEDITATION: Father God, I'm impressed! This covenant Jesus made for us is so strong that even He was raised from the dead by it. I imagine the devil hated His resurrection and fought to keep Jesus dead in the tomb. But You raised Him by Your Spirit through this eternal covenant. This covenant has resurrection power. This covenant defies the devil. The devil can't annul this covenant. Your covenant with me is eternal, not temporary. This covenant is forever sure, signed in blood by Jesus, who never lies. My healing is a sure thing. Praise God!

✞ ✞ ✞

There's more. What is the Eucharist and why is there power in it? Would you pray with me that we experience more of the power of the covenant meal?

Chapter 21

God Heals You Through the Eucharist (Holy Communion)

There is power in the Lord's Supper. In reading the Scriptures below, no one can doubt the power involved. If there is power to make sick, there is also power to make well. If there is power to cause death, there is also power to create life.

Some call it "communion," others, "the Eucharist." No matter what term you use, Christ designed it for *an experience with Him*.

Long-time church members have read these scriptures and heard them preached many times. I was no exception. Frankly, communion and the verses relating to this sacrament didn't mean a whole lot to me. I just went and took communion like everyone else. But somehow, I had a hidden feeling there had to be more to it than I was experiencing.

I'm sorry I had to learn in a backward way, but this is how it happened for me. At our church we "celebrated" communion once a month. Every month the same. Occasionally, I got headaches. Inconvenient, but nothing too serious. But why the headaches? After two or three headaches of unknown cause, I realized they followed communion. I wasn't sure but didn't want to take chances. I asked God to show me if the headaches were caused by something related to the bread and wine.

What came to mind was an eye-opener. I realized there was a person who had offended me years earlier whom I had not forgiven. Immediately, I forgave in my heart. Did I ever get another "communion headache?" No, never! And that was the way God trained me. There is power in the Eucharist!

The Eucharist is rooted in the Passover meal that God initiated through Moses. The Passover meal took place just hours before the Exodus from Egypt. Can you imagine the condition of the Israeli people? They were slaves, harassed and whipped by merciless slave masters. But they ate the Passover Lamb, a representative of Jesus, the Lamb of God. Psalm 105:37 relates the powerful result of eating the Passover Lamb!

✞ ✞ ✞

Psalm 105:37 Then He brought them out with silver and gold, And among His tribes there was not one who stumbled. (NASB)

37 Then he led the Israelites out; they carried silver and gold, and all of them were healthy and strong. (GNT)

37 And he brought them forth with silver and gold; And there was not one feeble person among his tribes. (ASV)

37 And he brought them forth with silver and gold, and there was not one sick person among their tribes. (JUB)

37 He brought them forth also with silver and gold: and there was not one feeble person among their tribes. (KJV)

37 He brought the people of Israel out of Egypt. The Egyptians loaded them down with silver and gold. From among the tribes of Israel no one got tired or fell down. (NIRV)

37 He brought out Israel, laden with silver and gold, and from among their tribes no one faltered. (NIV)

MEDITATION: O Lord, I am moved by the power of the Lamb! The Passover Lamb was for the healing of the nation! You gave strength and healing to every feeble person in one night!

O Lord, You have brought me out of the old life of bondage to sin and sickness. You have chosen to give me health and abundant finances. All the blessings of heaven that You have for me, I now claim. I am healed today. My feet shall not slip, slide, nor stumble. I shall go on from faith to faith, from strength to strength, and from glory to glory. I shall enter into every one of your "land of promises" and find my inheritance there!

✞ ✞ ✞

1 Corinthians 11:30 For this reason many among you are weak and sick, and a number sleep [margin: are dead].

30 For this cause many are weak and sickly among you, and many sleep. (KJV)

30 That [careless and unworthy participation] is the reason many of you are weak and sickly, and quite enough of you have fallen into the sleep of death. (AMP)

30 Because of this violation, many in your community are now sick and weak; some have even died. (VOICE)

MEDITATION: O Lord, I'm regarding this with extreme seriousness. I encounter You in all Your power. I have repented of every known sin. If there is more, convict me. I have forgiven wherever there is need. Now I trust You to empower me to life, health, and Godly living. I believe You are making me well and whole through this communion with You. I am forgiven and healed through You. You are now in me and I am in You.

✟ ✟ ✟

Mark 14:22 While they were eating, He took some bread, and after a blessing He broke it, and gave it to them, and said, "Take it; this is My body."

1 Corinthians 11:24 and when He had given thanks, He broke it and said, "This is My body, which is for you; do this in remembrance of Me."

24 And when he had given thanks, he brake it, and said, Take, eat: this is my body, which is broken for you: this do in remembrance of me. (KJV)

24 The Master, Jesus, on the night of his betrayal, took bread. Having given thanks, he broke it and said, This is my body, broken for you. Do this to remember me. (MSG)

1 Corinthians 11:26 For as often as you eat this bread and drink the cup, you proclaim the Lord's death until He comes.

26 For as often as ye eat this bread, and drink this cup, ye do shew the Lord's death till he come. (KJV)

26 For every time you eat this bread and drink this cup, you are representing and signifying and proclaiming the fact of the Lord's death until He comes [again]. (AMP)

26 ... you reenact in your words and actions the death of the Master. (MSG)

26 ... you are retelling the message of the Lord's death, that he has died for you. (TLB)

MEDITATION: O Lord, I am proclaiming Your crushed and broken body for my healing. I was healed by Your stripes. Your broken body brought my healing. By taking Your broken body, I proclaim to myself and everyone else, "I'm healed by Jesus' wounds!"

I'm remembering Your lashes and wounds. I'm focusing on Your stripes. I'm concentrating on and meditating on Your broken, beaten, striped body. Your death liberated me from sin, sickness, guilt, shame, and the power of the devil!

I'm reenacting Your death and resurrection in my own body and announcing it to the world. My body is Your temple and You are glorified in me. I'm proclaiming Your resurrection life now in my own physical body. You are alive in me and I in You. No power of darkness can hold me down. Hallelujah!

✞ ✞ ✞

Some of us have to learn the hard way. My wife tells me I'm high-strung, and she's right. I tend to be a workaholic. When we were building our house, I used to exhort our boys, "Find a way to finish it today." I wanted every project completed *ex post haste*. A pet peeve of mine is the person who seems to live by the mantra "Never do today what you can put off 'til tomorrow."

What I didn't know is that stress contributes to cancer and other "diseases."

Chapter 22

God Heals You Through Peace

Dr. Dean Ornish, a pioneer in healing heart disease through lifestyle changes, has shown conclusively through scientific research that even severe heart disease can be stopped or reversed without medication.

These lifestyle changes focus on four areas: a low-fat diet including fruits, vegetables, whole grains, and legumes; walking or other moderate exercise; meditation or some other type of stress management/anxiety reduction; and to top it off, old-fashioned love and community support.

Stress reduction contributes to health and physical healing. The evidence is so strong that Medicare coverage began January 1, 2010 for qualified patients using Dr. Ornish's program.

I'm thankful for Dr. Ornish, his pioneering research, and his excellent program. He has documented what many believers have experienced for centuries.

Biblical peace, however, is greater than stress reduction. Simply reducing tension can leave a person empty and vulnerable to the next set of stressful circumstances or even diabolical attacks. The peace that Jesus Christ offers is a fullness of the nature of God Himself. Jesus offers an impartation of rest, assurance, confidence, and security that replaces tension and its physical and emotional symptoms. Biblical peace is not merely the absence of war; rather, it is wholeness and total well-being—physical, financial, emotional, and spiritual—based in Christ.

Jesus promised peace (stress reduction plus the very wholeness of God Himself) through the following words found in Scripture.

✞ ✞ ✞

Ephesians 2:14 For He Himself is our peace …

14 For he is our peace … (KJV)

Isaiah 9:6 For a child will be born to us, a son will be given to us; And the government will rest on His shoulders; And His name will be called Wonderful Counselor, Mighty God, Eternal Father, Prince of Peace.

9:6 Prince of Peace (KJV, AMP, VOICE, RSV, ESV, HCSB, DRY)

Isaiah 26:3 The steadfast of mind You will keep in perfect peace, because he trusts in You.

3 Thou wilt keep him in perfect peace, whose mind is stayed on thee: because he trusteth in thee. (KJV)

3 A person whose desire rests on you, you preserve in perfect peace, because he trusts in you. (CJB)

3 You will guard him and keep him in perfect and constant peace whose mind [both its inclination and its character] is stayed on You, because he commits himself to You, leans on You, and hopes confidently in You. (AMP)

Romans 5:1 Therefore, having been justified by faith, we have peace with God through our Lord Jesus Christ.

1 Therefore being justified by faith, we have peace with God through our Lord Jesus Christ. (KJV)

1 Having been declared righteous, then, by faith, we have peace toward God through our Lord Jesus Christ. (YLT)

1 Therefore, since we have been declared righteous by faith, we have peace with God through our Lord Jesus Christ. (HCSB)

Psalm 46:10 Cease striving and know that I am God; I will be exalted among the nations, I will be exalted in the earth.

10 Be still, and know that I am God: I will be exalted among the heathen, I will be exalted in the earth. (KJV)

10 Let go of your concerns! Then you will know that I am God. I rule the nations. I rule the earth. (GW)

10 Be still, be calm, see, and understand I am the True God. I am honored among all the nations. I am honored over all the earth. (YLT)

John 14:27 Peace I leave with you; My peace I give to you; not as the world gives do I give to you. Do not let your heart be troubled, nor let it be fearful.

27 Peace I leave with you, my peace I give unto you: not as the world giveth, give I unto you. Let not your heart be troubled, neither let it be afraid. (KJV)

27 Peace I leave to you; my peace I give to you, not according as the world doth give do I give to you; let not your heart be troubled, nor let it be afraid; (YLT)

27 I leave behind with you—peace; I give you my own peace and my gift is nothing like the peace of this world. (PHILLIPS)

27 I give you peace, the kind of peace that only I can give. It isn't like the peace that this world can give. So don't be worried or afraid. (CEV)

27 I am leaving you with a gift—peace of mind and heart. And the peace I give is a gift the world cannot give. So don't be troubled or afraid. (NLT)

Isaiah 57:19 … Peace, peace to him who is far and to him who is near," says the LORD, "and I will heal him."

19 I create the fruit of the lips; Peace, peace to him that is far off, and to him that is near, saith the LORD; and I will heal him. (KJV)

19 The LORD says, "Peace, peace to the one who is far or near, and I will heal him." (HCSB)

19 I will give peace, real peace, to those far and near. And I will heal them, says the Lord. (ICB)

19 I offer peace to all, both near and far! I will heal my people. (GNT)

19 "… Peace, peace, to those far and near," says the LORD. "And I will heal them." (NIV)

MEDITATION: Lord, I need Your help to settle down. I need Your grace to relax and let go. I bring my old self to the cross. I repent of my self-activity, my self-effort, and my dead works. I declare myself dead to sinful self and alive to God in Christ.

Help me to know deeply that I am accepted in the Beloved. Let me know afresh today You love me whether or not I perform or accomplish goals. You accept me as I am in Christ Jesus. Thank you.

I am righteous in You. You have declared me righteous in Your sight for all eternity. It is enough. Thank You.

I now accept Your peace and presence. I am letting Your peace roll over me like gentle waves in a river. You are all I need. I accept Your healing presence. I feel Your rest.

☦ ☦ ☦

God is making known His boundless desire to heal. He wants to heal us more than we want to be healed. For some, it's easier to pop a pill than to sustain our will to be healed by God. We may need to increase our motivation for spiritual healing. One of the most powerful motivations to receive healing is God's love and compassion.

Chapter 23

God Heals You Through Love and Compassion

The Bible word for compassion (in the original Greek language) is *splanchnizomai*, pronounced splangkh-nid'-zom-ahai. By definition it means to have the bowels yearn, i.e. (figuratively) feel sympathy, to pity; to be moved with compassion; to be moved as to one's bowels, have compassion (for the bowels were thought to be the seat of love and pity).

To say Christ "had compassion" means He was moved in the innermost part of His being. It means the core of his personality was shaken and revealed. It means "His heart was broken." Since the fullness of the God of love dwells in Jesus in bodily form, we can say, "The heart of the God who heals was exposed and released." That Jesus had compassion is to say, "The totality of the God of love and pity was flowing out through Jesus."

✟ ✟ ✟

Matthew 14:14 When He went ashore, He saw a large crowd, and felt compassion for them and healed their sick.

Matthew 20:34 Moved with compassion, Jesus touched their eyes; and immediately they regained their sight and followed Him.

Mark 1:41 Moved with compassion, Jesus stretched out His hand and touched him, and *said to him, "I am willing; be cleansed."

Luke 7:13-15 When the Lord saw her, He felt compassion for her, and said to her, "Do not weep." And He came up and touched the coffin; and the bearers came to a halt. And He said, "Young man, I say to you, arise!" The dead man sat up and began to speak. And Jesus gave him back to his mother.

13 And when the Lord saw her, he had compassion on her, and said unto her, Weep not. (KJV)

13 When the Lord saw her, his heart went out to her and he said, "Don't cry." (Phillips)

13 When the Lord saw the woman, he felt sorry for her and said, "Don't cry!" (CEV)

13 And having seen her, the Lord felt-deep-feelings [of compassion] for her. And He said to her, "Do not be weeping". (DLNT)

13 When Jesus saw her, his heart broke. He said to her, "Don't cry." (MSG)

13 When the Lord saw her, his heart went out to her and he said, "Don't cry." (NIV)

A brief look at theology helps us understand how God's love and compassion lead to healing.

Romans 5:8 But God demonstrates His own love toward us, in that while we were yet sinners, Christ died for us.

Romans 5:12 Therefore, just as through one man sin entered into the world, and death through sin, and so death spread to all men, because all sinned.

Romans 5:17 For if by the transgression of the one, death reigned through the one, much more those who receive the abundance of grace and of the gift of righteousness will reign in life through the One, Jesus Christ.

The thought process is clear: Just as Adam's sin brought certain automatic results, e.g., universal sin, so Christ's death brought certain results, e.g., righteousness and healing by His stripes. *He Himself bore our sins in His body on the cross, so that we might die to sin and live to righteousness; for by His wounds you were healed* (1 Peter 2:24). Yet each man must receive the grace God offers.

Let's say it again in another way: Christ's death for us—His demonstrated love—brought forgiveness of our sin. Jesus' death for us—His demonstrated love—brought abundance of grace to us. His death for us—His demonstrated love—brought the abundance of the gift of righteousness [justification] to us. The death of the Lord Jesus Christ—His demonstrated love—brought healing to us. We can say, "His love-stripes healed us," and "His love-wounds cured us." Or we can simply say what Peter said, "By His stripes we were healed" (1 Peter 2:24).

God demonstrated his love for us by His death. His death gained eternal righteousness for our souls. His "death stripes" gained healing for our bodies. His "love wounds" brought us the healing we need. Abundant grace is ours to receive His great salvation. Praise God!

MEDITATION: O Lord Jesus, You are the same today as You were on earth. Your compassion brought healing then. As I meditate, I feel Your compassion more and more. Your heart is broken over my sin and my sickness. Your heart is going out to touch me right now. I'm being healed by your love.

You are longing to heal. It is Your great pleasure to heal.

All that You are and have, You are giving to me. You died for me in love; You paid the price for my body in love. You are moved in Your innermost being to bring healing in me. I receive You now and I praise You.

How powerful is Your love! How great is Your compassion. Your love and pity for us are not "add-ons" to Your character; rather, they define who You are and always will be.

Your love carries us across the threshold from sickness to health!

✝ ✝ ✝

Epilogue and Concluding Thoughts

I'm Happy and Thankful to Be Alive

Toward the end of 2011 I began feeling the pains and numbness that led to the cancer diagnosis. Eventually, I nearly died two different times and was reduced to a near vegetative state. That all seems so long ago.

Today I am vibrant and well. Tests indicate no cancer. (I still have some symptoms in my feet—I can't play basketball yet—and expect those conditions to be healed also.) I feel good and work full time. I can walk, drive, swim, jump off a rope swing into our pond, and ride a bicycle. Chopping wood is my favorite exercise.

I thank God and many others for good health today. Each of the nine keys detailed in this book contributed to my recovery. The purpose of *Answer for Cancer: 9 Keys* is simple. I wrote to help you get well and stay healthy.

As I searched for healing, I had to learn new ideas. Without new approaches to life and health, I would be dead today.

Healing Often Requires New Concepts

Knowing God brings healing. We can't get healed by God without knowing Him and we can't know Him without getting some healing. Knowing God is healing in the fullest sense—spiritual, physical, and emotional. Healing is hidden in the nature of Him who loves us and died for our great salvation. Our salvation includes healing and health.

Some are seeking healing but not seeking God. That's taking a shortcut and it doesn't work very well. Some are seeking God but neglecting the natural elements. It doesn't always work that way either. This book emphasizes both the natural and the supernatural. I have put together nine natural and spiritual keys that contributed to the defeat of cancer in my life. The keys worked for me and they can work for anyone.

Healing necessitates acquiring new concepts. It is not an isolated event. Rather, healing is part of the great redemptive process during which God removes the cocoon of the old life and metamorphoses a believer into a new creature in Christ. To get healed we most likely need new ways of thinking.

Healing begins on the inside, in the spirit. It often starts small, small as a pin prick or seed. I'm convinced many people are healed and don't know it yet! If you are healed, act like you're healed!

Let's think about miracles. God uses natural substances to bring supernatural results. Ezekiel prophesied about the trees, that *their fruit will be for food and their leaves for healing* (Ezekiel 47:12). Jesus multiplied five loaves and two fish to feed five thousand men at one time. God can take natural substances such as vegetables and medicine, mix them with faith, and bring supernatural results. Is that not a miracle?

We may need a new way of thinking about the Bible. Does healing always need to be instantaneous? Are gradual healings supernatural also? Yes, of course. My own healing has been a series of both gradual and instantaneous events.

We may need a fresh look at faith. God's word is His medicine. "Just take your medicine; faith will be there when you need it." Faith is never static. Faith grows. Faith *comes* through Jesus Christ. I repeat, faith *comes* through Jesus.

Have you received Jesus Christ into your life? Here's the good news. Jesus Christ died for our sins; Jesus Christ rose again from the dead. He is offering the free gift of salvation to all who put child-like trust in Him. If you've not done it before, receive Him into your life now.

We may need to re-evaluate our personal role in healing. Personal responsibility is crucial. When my wife and I realized chemotherapy could not heal me, I had to find what it would take to survive. I found a health coach, I began to meditate on powerful healing Scriptures, and I changed my diet. It was nearly too late, but I finally took responsibility for my own health.

All healing is from God. Yet we need to realize God generally heals unbelievers differently from believers in Christ. Unbelievers are readily healed by the faith of the minister or a prayer team. God simply wants to show Himself real to the unbeliever.

Many years ago a dedicated young doctor from New York mentioned, "In my practice I pray for my patients, but I don't see them healed." I asked, "Are you praying for believers or unbelievers?" "Believers," came his reply. "Start praying for the unsaved and you will see results," I responded.

But to those who are His born again children, He is zealous to develop His divine nature of trust, patience, and love in each one. From outsiders He expects little. Of His own children He expects more. Jesus said, "To whom much is given, much is required." As a loving Father, God places the responsibility *and the grace for healing* squarely upon the shoulders of His own children.

What about the local church? Most likely, we need to understand the local church's role in healing with fresh perspective. When the church is working right, there is nothing like it on earth. Local churches can take the time and have the patience to deal with natural causes of disease such as toxins, improper diet, lack of nutrition, and failure to exercise. A traveling evangelist or apostle generally doesn't have either the time or the relationship with people to deal with the natural elements of the healing process.

We need to understand the differences between pastoral healing in the local church and the evangelistic or apostolic healing ministries. The latter have the gifts and anointing for miracles. Most pastors do not.

I recently asked an apostle, Neil Silverberg, "How can we put together natural healing and the type of supernatural healing we read about in Jesus' ministry in the Bible?" He replied, "I recently gave an altar call for healing at a local church. The line extended clear out the door. But I couldn't help notice how obese many of the people were." Then he went on to explain, "That's the ministry of the local church—help people with natural causes and solutions. The apostle doesn't have the time to do this."

What about God? We may need to get new ideas of who He is and what He's really like—ideas that He is waiting and wanting to give. What helped me so much as I struggled to overcome cancer was to get to know more of God Himself. His very nature is healing. It's who He is. Again, fish swim, birds fly, God heals. Understanding the nature of God pulled me into Him with magnetic force. This revelation of the nature of God served like a wondrous, mysterious magnet to pull me through the dark places of wondering and doubt. This comprehension of God's nature came as a result of meditation.

To know God is to experience healing. I don't mean to know about God intellectually; rather, to know Him as one person knows another. To know God is to experience healing. I don't mean only to know Him as Savior from sin. Many good Christians know Him as Savior from sin but have not yet come to know Him as Healer from sickness. To know God is to experience healing. I mean to know and experience Him as Jehovah-Rapha, the Lord our healer.

One of the greatest experiences I've received in my bout with cancer is to realize *God's pleasure is to heal people*. This understanding really motivates me. I love to feel His pleasure. As I meditate on His "healing pleasure Scriptures," He draws me to Himself. His pleasure mesmerizes and woos me across the threshold from faith to greater faith. I love it! There is perhaps no greater incentive to press in to God for His healing touch.

Final Words

WHY DOES CANCER SO OFTEN RETURN AFTER TREATMENT? BECAUSE CONVENTIONAL TREATMENTS DO NOT KILL CANCER STEM CELLS. The root of the cancer, the circulating cancer tumor stem cells in the blood, are not killed. Only the daughter cells, the offspring of the cancer stem cells are killed.

Listen to Dr. Russell Blaylock, MD and retired neurosurgeon:

The trouble with chemotherapy, and conventional treatments, is they have no effect on the cancer stem cell. They only kill the daughter cells—the cells that are produced by them. So the tumor will shrink, and they'll claim success, but you haven't killed the stem cell. So it all just comes right back. And … it comes back infinitely more aggressive than it did before.[24]

OF ALL I AM LEARNING ABOUT CANCER, THIS FACT IS ONE OF THE MOST IMPORTANT. TO ANYONE YOU KNOW WHO SUFFERS FROM CANCER, IT IS WORTH THE PRICE OF THIS BOOK THOUSANDS OF TIMES OVER.

TRUMPET THE TRUTH AS YOU GIVE ANSWER FOR CANCER: *9 KEYS* TO SOMEONE YOU KNOW AND CARE ABOUT.

No matter where you are in your healing journey, meditate on the truths of "God Heals—It's His Pleasure to Heal You" found in Chapter 17 of this book. Nothing may be more enticing to the one suffering than to feel the pleasure of God in the healing process. Allow God to be God. Most likely,

---

[24] *The Truth About Cancer: A Global Quest* © 2015, TTAC Publishing, LLC, USA.

you will feel His pleasure before you begin to feel His healing. He died both to acquit us of our sins and to cause our diseases to quit affecting us. Certainly, He does not want His stripes to go unused, ignored, or wasted. When we begin to feel His pleasure in healing, we are drawn into the very heart of our God who loves to heal.

Postscript

Everyone should know that the "war on cancer" is largely a fraud.
—Linus Pauling, PhD, Two Time Nobel Prize Winner

Let's Start With a Three-Question Test

Question #1: What causes a cell to be cancerous?

Question #2: What is the 5-year "cure rate" of orthodox medicine, meaning what percent of their cancer patients are alive 5 years after diagnosis?

Question #3: What is the 5-year "cure rate" of several of the best-known natural cancer treatment experts?

Think about your answers before reading on.

Most people think that cancer is caused by DNA damage and that orthodox medicine is frantically searching for a cure for cancer.

Cancer is not caused by DNA damage. The definition of a cancer cell is a cell with low ATP energy (i.e., a low level of adenosine triphosphate). Only a very, very small fraction of DNA has anything to do with the creation of ATP energy.

The low ATP level is actually caused by microbes which are inside the cancer cells, generally *Helicobacter pylori*. This is an amazing microbe which can have 16 different sizes and shapes depending on the pH it is exposed to.

This microbe intercepts glucose as it enters the cancer cells and thus reduces the amount of glucose available to be converted into pyruvate. With less pyruvate the cell will create less ATP energy. (Of course, I am skipping many steps in this process.)

The International Cancer Research Foundation (ICRF) has developed more than 20 cancer treatments that revert the cancer cells into normal cells. How do they revert cancer cells into normal cells? They safely target and kill the microbes inside the cancer cells.

Killing cancer cells is "old school" but there is nothing wrong with things that can safely target and kill cancer cells (such as purple grape juice), but the new approach is to kill the microbes inside the cancer cells. This was first done in the 1930s but that technology was persecuted and shut down by the FDA and AMA. It has been restored, however, by the High RF Frequency Devices.

Let's Talk About Cure Rates

You probably think that orthodox medicine (e.g., the pharmaceutical industry, oncologists, the American Medical Association or AMA, etc.) has a 5-year cure rate for cancer patients of more than 50%. A "5-year cure rate" would mean, by definition, that 50% or more of their cancer patients are still alive 5 years after being diagnosed with cancer.

You probably think that the Food and Drug Administration (FDA) is not only doing its best to find cures for cancer, but is shutting down "quacks" who are pretending to cure cancer but in fact do not know how to cure cancer.

You probably think that the media is constantly looking for who has the best cure rates for cancer so the media's investigative journalists can keep the general public apprised of who has the most effective cancer treatments.

Are your assumptions correct? NO!

Cure rates are not an academic issue because you, the reader, may get cancer some day or you may know someone who gets cancer, such as a spouse or relative. Your very life, or the life of a friend of loved-one, may be on the line as you decide who is telling the truth about cancer research.

Choosing a cancer treatment is literally a life-and-death decision. The "cure rates" for different cancer treatments can range from 3% to 95% for the same type of cancer. So let's talk about cure rates.

First, what is the overall 5-year cure rate of the oncology profession according to their own statistics? In other words, what percentage of their patients are still alive 5 years after diagnosis?

Second, what was the cure rate of a South African immigrant who used nothing but purple grape juice to treat cancer?

The answer to the first question is this: the 5-year cure rate of orthodox medicine (e.g., oncologists) is 2.1%. In other words, in 97.9% of the cases, their cancer patients are dead within 5 years of diagnosis. See this article from the Oncology Journal.[25]

The answer to the second question is this: Johanna Brandt's cure rate was 100%. God designed the DNA for purple grapes so that they could cure cancer.

Orthodox medicine cannot cure cancer, yet the cure rate for Johanna Brandt, who did not have a single day of a single class in medical school, was 100%.

Johanna Brandt did not need to know how to cure cancer; Mother Nature knew how to cure cancer! And Mother Nature had put at least 12 chemicals in purple grape juice that can kill cancer cells.

The best way to survive cancer is to figure out what Mother Nature has already done.

Dr. William D. Kelley, DDS was a dentist turned natural medicine cancer researcher. He worked with more than 30,000 cancer patients using his protocol.

Dr. Kelley had a cure rate of 93% on his newly diagnosed cancer patients who had not had chemotherapy, radiation, or surgery!

Dr. Kelley was thrown in jail and later went to Mexico to treat cancer patients. Why did he go to jail? Because he used products to treat cancer which cannot be patented. Thus, the pharmaceutical industry and medical community had no interest in his treatments because they cannot make huge profits from treatments that cannot be patented. So they had him thrown in jail. They did not care that he had a 93% cure rate; his treatments were not profitable enough to satisfy their greed.

Dr. Kelly used cancer treatments designed by God, meaning Mother Nature, such as natural enzymes. These enzymes made the cancer cells visible to the immune system and the immune system cured the cancer. The enzymes were natural and could not be patented.

In other words, Dr. Kelly was not a medical doctor and he used natural medicine to achieve his 93% cure rate. Using Mother Nature is an unforgivable sin according to the AMA and the media. His cure rate was irrelevant. Dr. Kelley died on January 30, 2005 at the age of 79.

---

[25] http://www.burtongoldberg.com/home/burtongoldberg/contribution-of-chemotherapy-to-five-year-survival-rate-morgan.pdf

So Let's Talk About Today

Today, the instant someone hears the term "natural medicine" they immediately run out the door as fast as they can run. But they are running away from the only highly effective cancer treatments. Mother Nature is a lot smarter than any chemist.

Many people have cured their newly diagnosed cancer by using a very healthy diet and drinking a quart of carrot juice (with a little beet juice mixed in) every day. That is all they did.

In fact, if all cancer patients did that, instead of using chemotherapy, radiation and surgery, the "cure rate" for cancer in America would jump dramatically.

But who would make huge profits telling cancer patients to drink a quart of carrot juice, mixed with a little beet juice, every day, and eat a healthy diet? Certainly not the medical community and certainly not the pharmaceutical industry and media. Carrot juice and beet juice cannot be patented. Nor can a healthy diet be patented.

The general public is so brainwashed they think that God (i.e., Mother Nature) is too stupid to be a medical doctor! Never mind the fact that God designed 100% of the DNA of carrots, beets, and humans. Scientists only understand about 3% of human DNA after studying it since 1953!

Dr. Philip Binzel, MD had an 81% cure rate using liquid laetrile from apricots. He got liquid laetrile from Mexico. The Food and Drug Administration (FDA) tried to block the importation of liquid laetrile into the United States. Fortunately, Dr. Binzel's son was an attorney and the FDA was defeated in court.

Dr. Royal Rife, a microbiologist, had a 100% cure rate using electro medicine to kill microbes inside the cancer cells. The American Medical Association (AMA) tried to buy him out. Rife refused so the FDA shut him down and destroyed his lab and inventory!

Why haven't the state medical boards forced the doctors in their states to use Dr. Kelley's cancer treatments?

Why don't the health insurance companies pay for the medical expenses of the cancer patients who use Dr. Kelley's cancer treatments? It would save their members billions of dollars a year.

Why hasn't Congress passed a law forcing all medical professionals to use the cancer treatments of Dr. Kelley?

Why hasn't the President of the United States ordered the Veterans' Administration hospitals to use Dr. Kelley's cancer treatments?

The reason is that everyone is looking for the most profitable cancer treatments, not the most effective cancer treatments. And the pharmaceutical industry has the most profitable cancer treatments! And everyone wants to be fed by Big Pharma.

The Savior of the world described this level of brainwashing in two words: "whited sepulcher." The media paints the whitewash on the sepulcher (the general public only sees the whitewash) and thus the general public has no idea what is inside the sepulcher or that the sepulcher even exists! They can't see the bodies behind the television screen.

Running to their medical doctor, in many cases, is the right thing to do. But in other cases (i.e., in the case of almost all diseases), it is the wrong thing to do. Your doctor has no clue how to cure cancer, AIDS, Alzheimer's, Multiple Sclerosis, ALS, and many other diseases. But there are people who do know how to deal with all of these diseases using natural medicine.

What if the FDA opened a cancer treatment center that used all of the natural cancer treatments they have shut down and some that are common knowledge which they did not shut down? What would the cure rate of this clinic be on newly diagnosed cancer patients?

The cure rate would be 100%.

—Webster Kerr, Founder of the Independent Cancer Research Foundation and the CancerTutor website

Acknowledgements

My wife Kari prays regularly for me and constantly encourages me. Thanks, Kari, for your partnership in life, in ministry, in writing, and in publishing. You are faithful to me "in sickness and in health."

Our children—Andrew, Ethan, Anna, Samuel, Matthew, John, and Sarah—who have prayed for me and supported me in so many practical ways. You kept abreast of everything at home, church, and farm when I needed you most. Thanks also for driving me to and from the hospital or Cancer Care Center when I was too sick to drive.

The Church of the Living Water in Muscatine, Iowa—you guys are great and I love you all for standing with me as I fought cancer. Your faith and encouragement helped bring me through the dark days. I couldn't have done it without you. Special thanks to our elders, Tom Lee and Bernie Blaskowski. I will never forget your support and prayers.

Don Dutcher, you are an answer to prayer. When you came on board to edit, you relieved mega amounts of pressure from me. Seriously, trying to format puts so much stress on me that I feared it might cause cancer to erupt again—even while I'm writing about healing from cancer! Thanks, Don.

Special thanks go to healing ministries who have preceded me. Kenneth Hagin was the first as far as I know to identify God's word as medicine based on Proverbs 4:20ff. T. L. Osborne and Morris Cerullo imparted faith to me. Bobby and Rhonda Martz, Philip and Helen Stanley, Wayne and Carolyn Crooke—all friends—by your example and use of spiritual gifts of faith, miracles, and healings, you have encouraged me.

Thanks to Jim Gallegan, businessman from Portland, Oregon who demonstrated remarkable gifts of faith, healing, and miracles and encouraged me to do the same.

Dr. Tony Jimenez, MD, is a scientist, researcher and the founder and director of the Hope4Cancer Institute. I offer you high praise. Few doctors are able to integrate natural and spiritual medicine as well as you. This man is gentle and a pleasure to listen to.

I acknowledge Vaughn and Ellen Colebrook, founders of Miracle Ministries, who built my faith through instantaneous miracles before my eyes.

I give special thanks to The Christian Family Fellowship, the first (at least to my knowledge) to develop and publish the parallels between natural and spiritual medicine.

Henry W. Wright's *A More Excellent Way to Be in Health* should be read by everyone who needs relief from sickness. Get a copy. Wright shows clearly how natural and supernatural elements work together for health and healing.

Thanks to Dr. Feeley and the staff of the Cancer Care Center in Iowa City, Iowa. When we didn't know where to turn for help, we prayed and God directed us to you. Dr. Feeley is a gifted oncologist and true gentleman. He twice intervened in my life when I was near death.

Thanks to Mercy Hospital in Iowa City and to the Genentech Company (the manufacturer of Rituxan, a chemotherapy drug) for paying for a significant portion of my medical costs. Diagnosis and emergency intervention— the crown jewels of the medical establishment—have twice helped save my life from impending death due to cancer.

Cancer has a bad habit of returning following chemotherapy treatments. When this happened to me, I became confused and bewildered, not knowing where to turn. Enter Webster Kerr! You led me onto a path of healing and restoration through your website (http://www.CancerTutor.com) and emails. You gave us hope. You recommended other cancer coaches with whom I talked or emailed. You were the first to alert me to Bill Henderson. I am alive today, at least in part, because of you. Thank you!

Chemo treatments can deal deathblows to cancer tumors, but they cannot keep cancer from returning. When cancer returned with a vengeance, Kari and I searched and prayed diligently for a maintenance program to keep me alive. Our son Andrew gave us a copy of Bill Henderson's *How to Cure Almost Any Cancer at Home for $5.15 a Day*. This book became an answer to our prayers. Without becoming a vegetarian, I am following the basics of Henderson's protocol and plan to continue for the rest of my life. Thanks to this kind and gentle man for finding a better way to treat cancer.

Thanks to Starla Weichmann of Be Healthy Naturally. You helped me discover some likely causes of cancer. Your inexpensive tests and supplements saved us thousands of dollars.

Thanks to Dr. Keith Scott-Mumby for your contribution about parasites. We needed to know.

Dr. Darrel Wolfe, Doc of Detox, you have handled a delicate topic with humor and grace. Your article, "Spoiled Rotten," changed my entire concept of detoxification. I recommend you and your site to everyone who will listen.

David C. Jockers, you helped convince me of the seriousness of environmental toxins. I can't be so careless as to ignore the reality any longer.

Here's to a genuine pioneer, Dr. Dean Ornish, MD. You have paved the way for the world (including me) to see the scientific value of meditation and good old-fashioned love and support groups. As a Christian theologian and student of the Scriptures, I laud you!

Emma Seppälä, PhD, is Associate Director of the Center for Compassion and Altruism Research and Education at Stanford University. I thank you, Dr. Emma, for publishing the scientific evidence for the healing power of meditation. Very encouraging!

Dr. Jason Rowe, chiropractor—your gentle hands did their best to solve the riddle of my impaired feet.

Thanks to my parents, Rognar and June Anderson, from whom I caught a love for God and His word. The older I get, the more I appreciate the goodness of a solid Christian family background. Some values are best instilled when you grow up with them.

Additional Resources

Cancer no longer needs to be a dreaded disease. Hundreds of cures are available if a person discovers them soon enough. Here are some resources that I use or am acquainted with. I receive no financial profit from any of these resources.

Cancertutor.com: If you don't know where to start, start here.

I go to the Cancer Care Center associated with Mercy Hospital in Iowa City, Iowa. The hospital, doctors, and staff are an answer to our prayers.

Bill Henderson, founder of www.beating-cancer-gently.com, and my own mentor, has helped thousands of people survive cancer.

Ty Bollinger, CEO of *The Truth About Cancer: A Global Quest* video series features scores of oncologists, doctors, and researchers who are curing cancer without radiation, surgery, and chemotherapy. Ty is the author of the monumental resource *Cancer—Step Outside the Box* and numerous other books. You can order from CancerTruth.net.

www.hope4cancer.com is the website for one of the most gifted cancer-treating doctors of whom I am aware. "I welcome the challenge of bringing recovery to patients suffering from cancer, heart disease, and other degenerative diseases," states Dr. Tony Jimenez, MD.

Be Healthy Naturally, owned by Starla Weichman, has saved me thousands of dollars through her diagnostic tools. Be Healthy Naturally combines the best of ancient natural medicine along with the latest modern technology to design a customized plan of care for each individual.

www.breastcancerconqueror.com is the web address for Dr. Veronique Desaulniers. The 7 Essentials System™ is a complete and step-by-step course that shows you exactly how to prevent "dis-ease" and heal your body. "Dr. V" is herself a breast cancer survivor.

John and Karen Kummerfeld, my neighbors. John is a long-term cancer survivor. They are easy to talk with. Their forte is essential oils; they also know more about the dangers of environmental toxins than you will ever want to hear. Phone (563) 785-4916.

Church of the Living Water in Muscatine, Iowa helps people receive healing using natural and spiritual means. Come to www.livingwatermuscatine.com. (Disclosure: I serve as pastor of The Church of the Living Water.)

Joyce Meyer is an influential author, speaker, and charismatic minister. Her website is www.joycemeyer.org.

Founded by Dr. Randy Clark, Global Awakening is a teaching, healing, and impartation ministry with a heart for the nations.

Bethel in Redding, California provides multiple resources for healing including conferences, schools, and training.

I seriously considered traveling to the Budwig Center in Malaga, Spain for treatment. They provide a wealth of information regarding the Budwig Diet and much more, including a free 90-page ebook.

Consider Utopia Wellness, operated by Dr. Carlos M. Garcia, MD. He is a medically trained doctor who practices holistic medicine. Dr. Garcia is world-renowned for his ability to remedy Stage 4 cancer as well as treat HIV and other diseases. His book, *Cancer-Free: Your Guide to Gentle, Non-toxic Healing*, Fourth Edition, serves as a welcome resource for anyone who needs help with cancer. Garcia's website is www.UtopiaWellness.com. I have talked with them; they are friendly and available to help.

Go to the Navarro Medical Clinic website for information on how to tell if you have cancer or if your cancer treatment is working. Their HCG urine test costs only $55.00 US dollars at the time of this writing and is well-regarded by many alternative medical providers. An inexpensive kit good for several tests from the Joe Ball Company makes the test easy to use.

I drink Essiac Tea every day for its healing and cleansing properties. Information about Essiac abounds on the internet.

I take melatonin if I wake up in the night. It helps restore sleep. Numerous modern studies show surprising anti-cancer properties for melatonin. It costs close to nothing and is available at health stores and online.

Iodine supplementation has restored mind and body to numerous people according to medical research and patient testimonies. I take four drops daily as a preventative.

Grassfed lamb and grassfed beef contain strong cancer-busting CLA or conjugated linoleic acid. In one study, scientists added minute amounts of CLA to breast cancer cells growing in a Petri dish. By the eighth day, 93% of the cancer cells were dead! Disclosure: our family raises and sells grassfed lamb bundles.

Joseph Mercola has one of the best health websites on the internet. His newsletter is free.

Dr. David C Jockers, DC is young, practical, and colorful. He has the experience and information you need to overcome cancer or live a healthy lifestyle. www.drjockers.com is an outstanding website.

Larry of Essence of Life is a great guy who has helped thousands of cancer patients. He is available by phone and will even return your call and talk with you. In my hour of need he answered one of my questions that has helped every day of my life. His website is a great source of information and products. Call (800) 760-4947 to talk with Larry or order products.

NOTE: While these additional resources may be helpful, no one should disregard the spiritual element. Cancer therapy books commonly cover everything from Ayurveda to Zinc but fail to consider God and prayer. *Answer for Cancer: 9 Keys* is different. This book covers a range of essentials and concentrates on the most powerful of all—connection with Jesus Christ the Redeemer and the God of the universe.

Permissions

21st Century King James Version (KJ21) Copyright © 1994 by Deuel Enterprises, Inc.; American Standard Version (ASV) Public Domain; (AMP) Amplified Bible Copyright © 1954, 1958, 1962, 1964, 1965, 1987 by The Lockman Foundation; Amplified Bible, Classic Edition (AMPC) Copyright © 1954, 1958, 1962, 1964, 1965, 1987 by The Lockman Foundation; Barclay, William Barclay's Daily Study Bible, 1956 Edition – Public Domain; (BBE) Bible in Basic English (1949/1964) -- Public Domain; Brenton Translation of the Septuagint -- Public Domain; BRG Bible (BRG) Blue Red and Gold Letter Edition™ Copyright © 2012 BRG Bible Ministries. Used by Permission. All rights reserved. BRG Bible is a Registered Trademark in U.S. Patent and Trademark Office #4145648; Common English Bible (CEB) Copyright © 2011 by Common English Bible; Complete Jewish Bible (CJB) Copyright © 1998 by David H. Stern. All rights reserved; Contemporary English Version (CEV) Copyright © 1995 by American Bible Society; Darby Translation (DARBY); Disciples' Literal New Testament (DLNT) Disciples' Literal New Testament: Serving Modern Disciples by More Fully Reflecting the Writing Style of the Ancient Disciples, Copyright © 2011 Michael J. Magill. All Rights Reserved. Published by Reyma Publishing; Douay-Rheims 1899 American Edition (DRA) Public Domain; EBR (Emphasized Bible) (Rotherham Bible) – Public Domain; Easy-to-Read Version (ERV) Copyright © 2006 by World Bible Translation Center; English Standard Version (ESV) The Holy Bible, English Standard Version Copyright © 2001 by Crossway Bibles, a publishing ministry of Good News Publishers; Etheridge -- Public Domain; Expanded Bible (EXB) The Expanded Bible, Copyright © 2011 Thomas Nelson Inc. All rights reserved; 1599 Geneva Bible (GNV) Geneva Bible, 1599 Edition. Published by Tolle Lege Press. All rights reserved. No part of this publication may be reproduced or transmitted in any form or by any means, electronic or mechanical, without written permission from the publisher, except in the case of brief quotations in articles, reviews, and broadcasts; GOD'S WORD Translation (GW) Copyright © 1995 by God's Word to the Nations. Used by permission of Baker Publishing Group; Good News Translation (GNT) Copyright © 1992 by American Bible Society; Goodspeed Bible texts credited to Goodspeed are from Smith and Goodspeed, The Complete Bible: An American Translation. Chicago: University of Chicago Press, 1931. 2nd edition, 1935; Holman Christian Standard Bible (HCSB) Copyright © 1999, 2000, 2002, 2003, 2009 by Holman Bible Publishers, Nashville Tennessee. All rights reserved; HNB (Holy Names Bible) Copyright 1963 by Scripture Research Association, All rights reserved; International Children's Bible (ICB) The Holy Bible, International Children's Bible® Copyright© 1986, 1988, 1999, 2015 by Tommy Nelson™, a division of Thomas Nelson. Used by permission; International Standard Version (ISV) Copyright © 1995-2014 by ISV Foundation. ALL RIGHTS RESERVED INTERNATIONALLY. Used by permission of Davidson Press, LLC; King James Version (KJV) by Public Domain; Leeser Bible Copyright: Tov Rose, Editor (Standard Copyright License); Lexham English Bible (LEB) 2012 by Logos Bible Software. Lexham is a registered trademark of Logos Bible Software; Living Bible (TLB) The Living Bible copyright © 1971 by Tyndale House Foundation. Used by permission of Tyndale House Publishers Inc., Carol Stream, Illinois 60188. All rights reserved; The Message (MSG) Copyright © 1993, 1994, 1995, 1996, 2000, 2001, 2002 by Eugene H. Peterson; Moffat: Bible: The James A. R. Moffat Translation Copyright 1922, 1924, 1925, 1926 by Harper Collins, San Francisco; Mounce Reverse-Interlinear New Testament (MOUNCE) The Mounce Reverse-Interlinear™ New Testament (MOUNCE) Copyright © 2011 by Robert H. Mounce and William D. Mounce. Used by permission. All rights reserved worldwide. "Reverse-Interlinear" is a trademark of William D. Mounce; Names of God Bible (NOG) The Names of God Bible (without notes) © 2011 by Baker Publishing Group; New American Standard Bible (NASB) Copyright © 1960, 1962, 1963, 1968, 1971, 1972, 1973, 1975, 1977, 1995 by The Lockman Foundation; New Century Version (NCV) The Holy Bible, New Century Version®. Copyright © 2005 by Thomas Nelson, Inc.; New English Translation (NET) NET Bible® copyright ©1996-2006 by Biblical Studies Press, L.L.C. http://netbible.com All rights reserved; New International Version (NIV) Holy Bible, New International Version®, NIV® Copyright ©1973, 1978, 1984, 2011 by Biblica, Inc.® Used by permission. All rights reserved worldwide; New International Reader's Version (NIRV) Copyright © 1995, 1996, 1998, 2014 by Biblica, Inc.®. Used by permission. All rights reserved worldwide; New King James Version (NKJV) Scripture taken from the New King James Version®. Copyright © 1982 by Thomas Nelson. Used by permission. All rights reserved; New Living Translation (NLT) Holy Bible. New Living Translation copyright© 1996, 2004, 2007, 2013 by Tyndale

House Foundation. Used by permission of Tyndale House Publishers Inc., Carol Stream, Illinois 60188. All rights reserved; New Revised Standard Version (NRSV) New Revised Standard Version Bible, copyright © 1989 the Division of Christian Education of the National Council of the Churches of Christ in the United States of America. Used by permission. All rights reserved; NHEB (New Heart English Bible) – Public Domain; Orthodox Jewish Bible (OJB) Copyright © 2002, 2003, 2008, 2010, 2011 by Artists for Israel International; J.B. Phillips New Testament (PHILLIPS) J. B. Phillips, "The New Testament in Modern English", 1962 edition by HarperCollins; Revised Standard Version (RSV) Revised Standard Version of the Bible, copyright © 1946, 1952, and 1971 the Division of Christian Education of the National Council of the Churches of Christ in the United States of America. Used by permission. All rights reserved; (RVR60) Scriptures marked as RVR60 are taken from the Reina-Valera 1960 version. Copyright © Sociedades Bíblicas en América Latina; Copyright © renewed 1988 United Bible Societies. Used by permission; The Voice (VOICE) The Voice Bible Copyright © 2012 Thomas Nelson, Inc. The Voice™ translation © 2012 Ecclesia Bible Society All rights reserved; Twentieth Century New Testament -- Public Domain; Wilson, Benjamin Wilson and the Emphatic Bible – not in copyright; World English Bible (WEB) by Public Domain. The name "World English Bible" is trademarked; Weymouth New Testament in Modern Speech Third Edition 1913 Public Domain--Copy Freely; Webster – Public Domain; Worrell, The Worrell New Testament (A. S. Worrell's Translation With Study Notes), copyright © 1904 by A. S. Worrell; copyright © assigned in 1980 to Gospel Publishing House, Springfield, Missouri; Wycliffe Bible (WYC) 2001 by Terence P. Noble; Young's Literal Translation (YLT) by Public Domain; J.B. Phillips New Testament

To contact the author or request a speaking engagement for your conference, college, church, or other organization, go to www.bmarkanderson.com.

Made in the USA
Columbia, SC
04 October 2017